Advance Praise for

"Better Humans is a must-read for all ages. Bernstein uses research and storytelling to illuminate the important truth that we are still in a pandemic—of mental health. *Better Humans* gives us a roadmap to get us through this crisis to a better place."

—**Eve Rodsky**, *NYT* Bestselling Author of
Fair Play and *Find Your Unicorn Space*

"I loved reading *Better Humans*! This book combines the elements of personal storytelling and informative statistics to educate and empower readers in a universal way—no matter who you are, I truly believe there is a story in this book that will resonate with you. Bernstein offers a reflective and thorough evaluation of what it has meant and continues to mean, to be human before, during and now after the pandemic, no matter your profession, experience, or identity. This book helped me reflect on how I hope to show up for my fellow humans, inspired by the variety of experiences I read!"

—**Dayna Altman MPH,** Mental Health Author, Entrepreneur,
Speaker at Bake it Till You Make it LLC, Participant in
MTV's 2022 Mental Health Youth Action Forum at The
White House with the Biden-Harris administration

"I was Janeane's fifth grade teacher and now the tables have turned. Janeane's thoughtful, empathic approach to today's mental health issues make her a great teacher who has important lessons for us all."

—**Nancy Schulman,** Senior Advisor,
Avenues The World School - Lifelong passionate educator;
Horace Mann School, 92nd Street Y Nursery School

"Janeane Bernstein's perspectives and dynamic interviews with students, teachers, and mental health professionals in her new book, *Better Humans*: *What the Mental Health Pandemic Teaches Us About Humanity*, is a must-read for those interested in a stimulating, compassionate, and empathic view of the global mental health pandemic. She interviews individuals who openly share their struggles, as well as mental health advocates and professionals who are working to scale mental health strategies and heal wounds that are often invisible. *Better Humans* provides a timely message of hope and empathy for humanity to learn and grow from the impact of the mental health pandemic."

—**Elaine Miller-Karas,** Co-Founder and Director
of Innovation of the Trauma Resource Institute

"Bernstein captures the current state of the mental health crisis in our society through research and storytelling. The book takes readers on a journey of reflection, and makes one want to be more self-aware of the energy people project into the world. Bernstein gives hope to the reader that better days are possible, but it is important to attend to our mental health and lean on one another."

—**Juan Acosta**, Mental Health + LGBTQ+ Activist,
Influencer, Speaker, White House Mental Health Youth
Action Forum Participant, *NYT* Bestselling coauthor

"Janeane Bernstein combines journalism's best talent for telling stories and contextualizing them with an advocate's desire to do more, as she reveals how the COVID pandemic exacerbated mental health issues too often ignored.

"To set the stage, *Better Humans* explains the background of mental health issues, the pandemic, how we arrived here, and where they intersect. The stories of *Better Humans* give the problems and solutions real texture and real-world context: mental health struggles and successes, and what is lost when we ignore them. They resonate because we know the people who live them—the teachers and nurses, the students, and the advocates. *Better Humans* brings them to us so we may learn how and why we must prioritize our mental health much like our physical health. This the core of *Better Humans*.

"You won't read *Better Humans* straight through once and put it on the shelf forgotten. You will read it first for knowledge and then again as a resource. Maybe you return to the stories as they call to you to help students grow into better humans themselves. Maybe you return to the resource list or the policy discussions to advance mental health support in your community. *Better Humans* is a long overdue call to action—for education, for compassion, for growth—to become better, healthier, humans."

—Hillary Sobel, Member of the Board of Directors of Right to Be (f/k/a Hollaback) New York City and Social Justice Advocate

"Better Humans is a call to action to prioritize mental health and well-being. The COVID-19 pandemic highlighted the importance of mental health and the ripple effects it can have on every aspect of our lives. Sharing insights and lessons learned from conversations with people of all ages, the book sheds a light on the root causes of depression and hopelessness, while also highlighting the positive aspects of learning new things, reconnecting with oneself and others, and prioritizing mental, physical, emotional, and spiritual health.

"Janeane aims to encourage readers to be more compassionate, empathetic and aware of mental health issues, as well as ending the stigma around discussing them by focusing on teaching people to be present, listen better, educate themselves on marginalized communities, embrace differences and to prioritize mental health in all aspects of society. Despite the challenges, there is an opportunity to create positive change, learn from the current situation and work towards healing the mental health pandemic.

—Sky Bergman, Filmmaker, Professor Emeritus of Photography and Video at California Polytechnic State University

Also by Janeane Bernstein, Ed.D.

Get the Funk Out!: %^&* Happens, What to Do Next!

BETTER HUMANS

WHAT THE MENTAL HEALTH PANDEMIC TEACHES US ABOUT HUMANITY

FOREWORD BY **ERIN RAFTERY RYAN**
Executive Director NAMI Westside Los Angeles

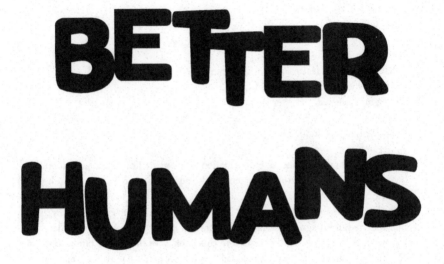

BETTER HUMANS

WHAT THE MENTAL HEALTH PANDEMIC
TEACHES US ABOUT HUMANITY

JANEANE BERNSTEIN, Ed.D.

Post Hill
PRESS

A POST HILL PRESS BOOK
ISBN: 978-1-63758-708-9
ISBN (eBook): 978-1-63758-709-6

Better Humans:
What the Mental Health Pandemic Teaches Us About Humanity
© 2023 by Janeane Bernstein, Ed.D.
All Rights Reserved

Cover design by Tiffani Shea

This book contains advice and information relating to health care. It should be used to supplement rather than replace the advice of your doctor or another trained health professional. You are advised to consult your health professional with regard to matters related to your health, and in particular regarding matters that may require diagnosis or medical attention. All efforts have been made to assure the accuracy of the information in this book as of the date of publication. The publisher and the author disclaim liability for any medical outcomes that may occur as a result of applying the methods suggested in this book.

Post Hill Press
New York • Nashville
posthillpress.com

Published in the United States of America
1 2 3 4 5 6 7 8 9 10

CONTENTS

FOREWORD

Dear Better Humans,

I hope this finds you well.

Ring! Ring! It's 2018, and I'm sitting in my office near the UCLA campus in Westwood, California. The phone rings. Yes, an actual landline phone. My reaction is to quickly answer the call, and yet I hesitate. My body tenses with a twinge of anxiety because of the uncertainty of what waits for me on the other end of the phone. It rings again. I take a deep breath, close my eyes, and prepare to provide support. "Hello, NAMI Westside Los Angeles, this is Erin, how can I help you? *(For those of you who know NAMI, you know! And for those of who don't, NAMI is the National Alliance on Mental Illness, which is the nation's largest grassroots organization dedicated to improving the lives of those affected by mental health conditions. So essentially, we are dedicated to helping everyone, as is the message in this amazing book!)*

Context. One in five U.S. adults and one in six U.S. youth aged six to seventeen experience a mental health disorder each year. Suicide is the second leading cause of death among people aged ten to fourteen. Millions of people in the U.S. are affected by mental health conditions each year. That means you or someone you know and love is affected. It's important to measure how common mental health conditions are, so we can understand their physical, social, and financial impact—and so we can show that no one is alone. These numbers are also powerful tools for raising public awareness, stigma-busting, and advocating for better health care. Many people don't know about the importance of mental health until they are in crisis and need answers. As the executive director of NAMI Westside

Los Angeles County, I have answered the phone many times to hear a sobbing mother, sister, husband, or friend on the other line reaching out for urgent help, feeling like there is nowhere to turn and they are all alone on this journey.

Feeling alone. That all started to change in 2020, when humanity experienced a collective trauma. Ring, ring…it's COVID-19, a global pandemic calling. Well, no one was prepared to answer that call! But in some capacity, we all had to deal with the unfathomable number of deaths, pervasive sense of fear, economic instability, and forced physical distancing from loved ones, friends, and our individual communities. This collective trauma exacerbated unprecedented stresses and—if there could be a silver lining—it also shed a new light on the importance of our collective mental health. The shame and stigma associated with mental health was put on hold and then put on speaker phone. The human race was experiencing feelings of isolation, anxiety, depression, and uncertainty from the pandemic, and we were in it together.

A call to action. On December 7th, 2021, a fifty-three-page advisory from U.S. Surgeon General Vivek H. Murthy focused the nation's attention on the youth mental health crisis. He states, "Our obligation to act is not just medical—it's moral. I believe that, coming out of the COVID-19 pandemic, we have an unprecedented opportunity as a country to rebuild in a way that refocuses our identity and common values, puts people first, and strengthens our connections to each other."

We have an opportunity to be better humans. My colleague and fellow heart leader, Janeane Bernstein, is answering the Surgeon General's call to action with her amazing work in the mental health space and most recently with her new book, *Better Humans*. And YOU are one of them. Kudos to you for reading this book!

You are a traveler on the life path of learning and growth. Prepare to be inspired by the heartfelt authentic stories of the previously untold silent battles with mental health and the voices of youth, our future leaders in this space. Get ready to be informed by what created and fueled the mental health pandemic and learn from the stories and insights of teachers, educators, and mental health professionals, often the ones on the frontlines of this pandemic. You will have the opportunity to think outside the box, hear from people of ages and backgrounds, and walk away with real time resources.

I first met Janeane as a guest on her podcast. She is a wonderful listener and storyteller and creates a safe space for truth to shine. She shares pure vulnerability and golden nuggets of wisdom throughout the book. Janeane's varied background in education, media, technology, teaching, communications, and journalism create an all-encompassing eclectic lens for the reader to gain perspective with tangible tools and candid conversations. Reading this book feels like you're having a cup of coffee with some of your dearest friends, reflecting on what happened and discussing, how can we be better? How can we do better for ourselves and others? These are big questions! And you are a better human for asking them. So happy to have shared a few words with you and have you join Janeane on her journey in finding solutions.

Be well, better humans.

With gratitude,
Erin Raftery Ryan
Executive Director
NAMI Westside Los Angeles

INTRODUCTION

*"Everyone you meet is fighting a battle you know
nothing about. Be kind. Always."*
—Robin Williams

I wanted to write *Better Humans* to share with you, my fellow humans, how we need to be better and do better as a collective whole. This book is for students, teachers, parents, school administrators, businesses, policymakers, and anyone else really, as I provide a glimpse into what you should know about the mental health pandemic, how we got here, and its impact. I have included numerous conversations with people of all ages who share lessons learned and insights into how you and I can be better to ourselves, our loved ones, colleagues, and total strangers. We need to do better as humans with the choices we make, how we take care of one another, and how we connect and communicate. We need to embrace diversity and inclusivity and prioritize and treat mental health and well-being.

We must examine each and every context and every possible demographic impacted by the lack of mental health services due to inequities, disparities, and inclusivity. We are a hurting nation where students' and adults' mental health needs are unmet. The wait time or access to mental health professionals is worrisome, and if you do manage to get an appointment, there is not enough time and resources to address the magnitude of needs. Without help, mental health issues impact every aspect of your life, causing a ripple effect of issues. Solutions and strategies are not happening soon enough, and the lack of attention and prioritization given to mental health became even more apparent from 2020 on. Now you and I have an opportunity to create a world that can positively impact the minds and actions of students of all ages, adults in every work setting and age group; this is the time to end mental health stigma in all contexts and change the trajectory of peoples' lives.

COVID-19 was a wake-up call for humanity and a test to our own resilience. I don't know very many people who haven't experienced some form of loss since March 2020; this loss might have been losing a friend or relative to COVID-19 or another illness, either suddenly or long-term. Losing yourself was a common theme as well, as more and more people sought psychological counseling for a new or past trauma, addiction, or mental health issue, while marginalized groups never had the support and resources to begin with. And the demand for mental health professionals outweighed availability and access.

Beginning in March 2020, you might have also lost your interpersonal connections, your job, your sense of self-worth, and felt disconnected from the very people under your roof, as you tried to process the news of the world. You were consumed with stress and anxiety as you tried to get through the long days. Days blended into weeks, months, and now years on Zoom. Your life consisted of multitasking as a mother, for example, trying to work from home, homeschool kids, pay bills, put food on the table, and maintain your sanity, all while grieving the loss of a loved one or several.

No one would have anticipated how 2020 would devastate millions of lives, within the United States and throughout the world. One day we are in crowded airports, traveling the world, visiting amusement parks, attending concerts, cheering our favorite teams in packed stadiums, having dinner with friends and colleagues, running through Grand Central Station in rush hour, visiting museums, going to the movies, partying on college campuses, and connecting physically and emotionally—shaking hands, hugging, kissing, chatting with strangers—and the next, life as we knew it was shattered.

We could not have fathomed that a virus that originated in Wuhan, China would devastate our world like a science fiction movie most of us would never want to see. In February 2020, I remember sitting in the aisle seat of an airplane next to a woman in the middle seat, who looked weak and feverish. She barely moved the entire flight, except for her head that flopped back and forth as she slept. I thought she might have bronchitis or the flu. For some reason, I had a surgical mask in my purse, and I thought, "I don't want to catch bronchitis (my kryptonite)," so I quickly put my mask on. When we landed, the woman to the right of her looked stressed and said to me, "She is so incredibly sick. That was so smart you wore a mask!" Little did I know, my seatmate might have had COVID-19, which was not even part of my vocabulary then.

Flash forward and millions of people lost their lives to COVID-19, experienced massive job losses, went through the mental and emotional effects of social isolation, witnessed and/or participated in protests, viewed senseless and horrific deaths from police brutalities, discrimination of all kinds, devastating school shootings and other unimaginable incidents of gun violence, massive disruption of supply chains, soaring rates of domestic violence, abuse, racial and ethnic inequities, homelessness, anxiety, depression, suicide, divorce, drug and alcohol abuse, consequences from isolation, struggles of working from home, including juggling work–life balance, food insecurity, and so on.

No one was immune to the ripple effects of the pandemic. I did have a conversation or two in 2020 with people who were living in their own little bubbles, not in touch with the reality and suffering of those affected by COVID-19; it pained me to listen to their insignificant miniscule "struggles." All I had to do was view the numerous emotional Instagram posts in 2020 from crying, exhausted, and terrified nurses who were brand-new to their field, and I felt their pain reverberate through me.

And then there were students, teachers, counselors, therapists, doctors, frontline workers, and more who openly shared an inside look at their daily emotional pandemic struggles that most of us would never go through. Millions of people lost jobs, looked for work that seemed impossible, or worked remotely in a whole new world of chaos. For those living in retirement homes, COVID-19 forced them into social distancing and isolation from loved ones to keep them safe, but the social isolation became detrimental to their mental, emotional, and physical health. Mothers and caregivers tried to manage all aspects of their lives under one roof—work, childcare, homeschooling, remote learning, motherhood, and other relationships all melded together like a weird new flavor of ice cream that no one had ever heard of (or wanted, for that matter).

There was no prep time to learn how to function remotely in social isolation. Schools had to shift rapidly to online instruction, and pandemic life replaced what was "normal" and familiar. Thus began a life of mental, physical, and emotional trauma that was adorned by masks of all types and a constant dose of hand sanitizer, social distancing, isolation, fear, and anxiety.

You might have been one of the millions of students having to live at home, no longer able to experience college life and the freedom of personal growth. You heard plenty of stories about how great college life was going to be, but yours was an experience confined to your bedroom staring at a computer screen. So, you chose to shut your computer cameras off during classes and became a faceless black screen with a name. Maybe you were paying attention, or doing something else like sleeping, eating, watching TikTok videos, or scrolling on your phone to just numb out your pandemic pain. You had to shut yourselves out from the world to the detriment of your mental, physical, and emotional health, and the plethora of suffering is not surprising.

As I set out to structure this book, there seemed to be more and more articles published about prioritizing mental health in schools and businesses, but what does this really mean? And when will there be a mental healthcare system that provides equal access, resources, and enough skilled professionals that offer training and education for diverse and difficult needs of people of all ages and backgrounds? With a shortage of trained therapists and counselors, you might have finally decided to reach out for help, only to find that you can't find anyone available, or your insurance doesn't cover therapy. If you reached out to your counseling center at your school, the wait times were long, and the resources limited; this was disheartening because how were you supposed to get the help you needed?

There must be consistent messaging about mental health, training and education, and an elimination of stigma. Mental health professionals must also be compensated properly for the essential work they do and the long, stressful days they face treating a wide variety of mental health issues and illnesses. The pandemic raised awareness around empathy, acceptance, a dismantling of mindsets, and the creation of policies and priorities that put mental health at the forefront. These are societal changes that will impact the trajectory of future generations. We can't afford to look away at the structural problems in the mental healthcare system, the exodus of essential workers, and the lack of initiatives to meet the needs of children and adults.

We needed mental health action a long time ago, but it took a pandemic to prove it. The media shines a light almost daily on how there are initiatives to reduce the stigma associated with mental health, and celebrities are speaking out as well. However, these conversations must be embedded in consistent messaging and agendas in our educational institutions, healthcare systems, and in the minds and actions of parents and other individuals throughout society so we are all on the same page reinforcing the same messages. Mental health initiatives must take precedent. You can be an incredible student academically, but if you are struggling with mental health issues and a drug addiction, you will face an uphill battle throughout your lifetime.

Mental health stigma and acceptance of the status quo is embedded in our culture. However, 2022 was a wake-up call to stop numbing out and do away with mindsets that are outdated and do not serve us. Our world is suffering. People of all ages, socioeconomic backgrounds, gender and racial identities, and professions are hurting, and the data proves it. The question is what can be done and how soon? We have lost touch with what really matters: human connection, thoughtfulness, empathy, compassion, intergenerational experiences, consistent and inclusive mental health initiatives that reach diverse and marginalized communities, and meaningful experiences that lift us up and bring people together instead of further dividing us.

Many of us are numb to the constant chaos and horrific news of more school shootings. As of October 5, 2022, *Education Week* magazine reported that there have been thirty-five school shootings in the U.S. resulting in deaths or injuries. These incidents are often caused by young men in their late teens and twenties. Where did the origins of all of this hate come from? Why would anyone decide to purchase assault rifles, boast about them on social media, and shoot up a school, killing teachers, staff, and innocent children, shortly after killing their grandmother? The U.S. has a serious gun problem, but at the root is also a mental health issue, where research is needed to study the backgrounds of the people who plan such horrific acts of violence. Their social media accounts need to be analyzed, and social media companies must be held accountable by reviewing accounts 24/7. They need to set standards for what is acceptable and not acceptable content and take action on red flag warnings. Right now, it feels like the Wild West and anything goes on social media, including sex trafficking, child porn, abuse, and hate crimes.

I believe some incidents of gun violence reflect a life lived in a cycle of abuse and suffering that perpetuated from childhood through adulthood. Oftentimes, these individuals suffer from mental illness, social rejection, depression, and abuse as children. With support from school administrators, teachers and staff should tune in to students who don't seem to fit in, such as social outcasts, or anyone else who seems troubled, and implement ongoing mental health and wellness check-ins with students. This can be done on an app every morning like you would when you seek mental health counseling. With well thought-out strategies for early detection in schools and work settings, only then will we begin to see a reduction in hate crimes, and people can get the care they need. People suffer in silence, and no one knows until it is too late.

Why didn't anyone notice the self-inflicted marks on the Uvalde, Texas shooter's face and do anything before he flipped a switch and destroyed lives May 2022? In an interview with *ABC News*, students said they were frightened of him. He boasted about the cut marks he did himself. Wasn't this enough of a red flag to do something? Who should have followed through, and what could have been done? This is now an all-too-common occurrence. Students are frightened to go to school—a place where they are not supposed to be having shooter drills and worried about whether their school is next. Schools are a place to interact, grow socially and emotionally, and feel safe and connected.

Is it any surprise that students are experiencing so much trauma, anxiety, depression, and so many suicidal thoughts? The weight of the world is too much and after having been forced to study remotely, many don't feel connected when they are finally back in person. We have lost our ability to connect, to feel connected, to feel heard and understood. Many don't feel listened to, and they might not have someone they can vent to, so they keep everything inside. They escape to their inner worlds and numb out. School staff and teachers are pushed to their limit. They not only shifted to online learning but dealt with ongoing debates on everything from mask policies to what should be taught in the curriculum (e.g., critical race theory), while being poorly compensated and disrespected.

Hundreds of thousands of teachers have left their profession. School mental health professionals and staff have not been properly trained and equipped to handle the growing demands of the pandemic; they left, too. However, when you hear from some of the young adults interviewed for this book, sometimes all someone wanted was someone to listen to whatever it is they were going through and for that listener to then share their own story of personal struggles, all without passing judgment. They just wanted to know there was someone available to connect with and to feel heard.

How are you? No, really. How are *you*? Truthfully, you might *not* be okay. Millions of people of all ages are filled with anxiety, depression, suicidal thoughts, PTSD, and more. We are numbing out on TikTok, Instagram, and other platforms. There is a spike in substance abuse for numerous reasons, ranging from depression and anxiety to someone's life completely imploding and not feeling seen and heard. There are also long-term effects of COVID-19. Many people have had COVID-19 on more than one occasion, and long-term side effects can zap you of your energy, mentally deplete you, and spiral you into despair. Sadly, people share on social media their raw emotions, pain, and suffering and how their life has been put on hold because of the long-term effects of this deadly virus, which was once not even part of our vocabulary back in early 2020.

People have spent an enormous amount of time socially isolated, making being back in person awkward and uncomfortable. We have forgotten how to communicate. We are tethered to our electronic devices, which provide comfort and a lifeline to other places to retreat to mentally and emotionally. Another downside to our tech addiction is that we see things we will never be able to unsee. Images and news are available 24/7 that are often graphic and amped up to feed the media machine, getting people to click and view on images not meant for consumption. No wonder we are up at night scrolling, swiping, looking for something that will make us feel whole but at the same time feeling hopeless, disengaged, and filled with feelings of inadequacy and unfulfillment, unable to feel gratitude for what is right in front of us.

Where would we have been without Zoom and Google Meet? I am thankful for our technology, but we are inundated with so much information and creators posting millions of images and videos all vying for our attention, a lot of times designed to be "clickbait." What we see on social media can oftentimes be detrimental to our psyches and self-esteem, and the addiction to creating and keeping up with everyone else is an exhaustive beast.

While technology has connected us in a time of enormous disconnect, it has also harmed the mental health of so many, especially those in the Generation Z age group. There is pressure to act and look a certain way, capture moments of the minute details and private moments of our days, and buy certain products, clothes, and other items that will make you even more attractive because it seems you are not attractive enough. You are neither thin nor pretty, handsome, or cute enough. You need to have a filter on when you post. We live in a more amped-up world of comparing ourselves constantly, negating ourselves, obsessing over total strangers we see online and aspiring to the images they portray, which is most likely an illusion.

The messages on social media have polluted us. "Buy this, buy that, and you can look as amazing and be as popular as me." Let's face it, people are exhausted mentally, physically, and emotionally; we are looking to feel better in a time of immense turmoil and polarization. Many of us are numb to the horrific news about school shootings, suicide rates, depression, and hopelessness. Life is no longer about "getting good grades and getting into a great school." Life means more to so many people, and it should. If we don't prioritize mental health in K–12, and in every aspect of society, where will students be in college and through adulthood? There has never been such chaos as there is now. People need to feel heard and shift what really matters in their lives. If you are fortunate enough to have spent time visiting a place you seldom visited (your true thoughts and feelings), welcome to an enlightened time. During the past few years, you experienced an incredible and surprising journey of self-discovery, a time of personal insight into what and who matters in your life and what and who doesn't, and you have learned who lifts you up, listens to you, and who doesn't.

Through all the tumult of the pandemic, the stories shared in this book illuminate everything from pandemic and online burnout to the root causes of depression and hopelessness. There are also bright spots in learning new things, reconnecting with oneself and others, and taking better care of our mental, physical, emotional, and spiritual health. Moving out of our comfort zone and trying new activities were also a theme in the pandemic; these are skills that can be transformative throughout your lifetime.

If there is anything you can learn from this pandemic, it is that peeling back your layers is essential to discovering who you really are, seeing your current and past struggles, facing your mental health and wellness challenges, learning about your interests and aspirations, and overcoming obstacles that prevent you from taking the very best care of yourself. Tune into yourself, your family, friends, colleagues, teachers, complete strangers, and anyone in your life, because "going back to normal" and "the way things used to be" is no longer an option. Amping up your level of thoughtfulness, empathy, and compassion will enable you to tune in to what really matters: the life you truly want to live and who you want along for the ride.

CHAPTER 1

The Mental Health Crisis – The Silent Battle

*"I was trying to express I was struggling.
I was trying to express that I could tell there was something wrong,
and I would often just get blamed for it. I wasn't good with time
management.I wasn't good with impulse control. I wasn't good.
I later found out I have ADHD. I grew up not getting the support
I needed as a neurodivergent person who has very extreme
anxiety, and self-soothing techniques that I created for myself."*
—Rocket Garcia, 24

People have been suffering with mental health issues for centuries. Some people struggle their entire lifetime, and all it takes is something unexpected, like a pandemic or other life-changing event, to stir up just how much they have silently and painfully suppressed. However, it is never too late to address a mental health issue, especially if it has held you back from thriving and you have felt the subject is just too taboo to talk about. The only problem is that there needs to be a mental healthcare system that is available to everyone, openly accepting, and with well-trained and educated staff and resources in place to meet the demand. Imagine that.

Cultural acceptance and attitudes around mental health have influenced opinions and policymakers. If you suffer in silence, you might not have the knowledge, support, resources, or resilience to pull yourself out of a spiraling life filled with depression, hopelessness, addiction, anxiety, and more. Some of us hide our problems better than others, but when unforeseen circumstances occur, you just never know what someone will reveal. Oftentimes, this can be a post-traumatic incident that was tucked away like a Pandora's box.

What is mental health? According to the World Health Organization (WHO), "Mental health is a state of mental well-being that enables people to cope with the stresses of life, realize their abilities, learn well and work well, and contribute to their community. It is an integral component of health and well-being that underpins our individual and collective abilities to make decisions, build relationships and shape the world we live in. Mental health is a basic human right. And it is crucial to personal, community and socio-economic development." Mental health is different for everyone, and factors such as biology, environment, and how we process the daily stressors and challenges of life affect us differently.[1]

Mental health encompasses your psychological, social, and emotional well-being and affects your thoughts, feelings, and actions. How you handle stress, your reactions to life events, and your relationships are all influenced by mental health. When the world was ravaged by COVID-19, any pre-existing problem you had might have been exacerbated, and more issues followed suit. The pandemic created a multitude of personal and professional struggles, and millions of people of all ages, ethnicities, gender identities, and socioeconomic backgrounds experienced loss, trauma, and uncertainty. These traumatic life experiences led to an increased need for mental health services that were not readily available to everyone, especially marginalized communities. As the demand for mental

---

[1]   World Health Organization, "Mental health: strengthening our response," June 17, 2022, https://www.who.int/news-room/fact-sheets/detail/mental-health-strengthening-our-response.

health professionals increased, a shortage of qualified counselors and therapists made life more challenging.

In writing this book, I turned to my daughter, who struggled significantly before and at the beginning of the pandemic. She is now a twenty-year-old college student, majoring in psychology. I asked her why she thought we were in a mental health crisis before the COVID-19 pandemic began. Her responses made me pause and consider the fact that many adults do not know what it is like to be Generation Z in a pandemic or to be someone who is struggling with a mental illness. She made several important points about the mental health crisis prior to 2020:

- There were misconceptions and a lack of training and education on what mental health struggles look like.
- People didn't know how to diagnose mental health struggles (e.g., school staff, therapists, counselors).
- There was no proper treatment.
- The people who struggled were afraid to speak up because of stigma and shame.
- People who struggle might not have supportive parents, and they might not feel understood.
- People who struggle might not have the support they need at all.

I then asked my daughter to fill in the blanks on the following statement:

People who struggle with mental health issues feel _____ and _____.

Her response was:

People who struggle with mental health issues feel <u>alone</u> and <u>misunderstood</u>.

She said other possible answers could be hopeless, anxious, depressed, unseen, or lonely. As a parent, I just sat with her responses for a bit and let them sink in, asking myself what it must feel like to live with these feelings before and during the pandemic. My heart was heavy not just for her, but for anyone really.

Biology, environmental factors, life circumstances, and the choices you make can also affect your mental health. This includes genetics, family history, traumatic childhood experiences (see ACES or Adverse Childhood Experiences assessment)—and even problematic societal issues such as violence, inequities, discrimination, and poverty play a significant role.

Prior to the pandemic, mental health struggles might have been exacerbated by some of the following:

- Pre-existing mental health conditions
- Lack of attention to mental health struggles
- Racial disparities with regards to who can receive mental health care
- Unhealthy home life (lack of food, abuse, unhealthy relationships, etc.)
- Lack of sleep
- Tech addiction
- Decreased physical activity
- Substance abuse
- Stress, anxiety, and depression
- Post-traumatic experiences
- Discrimination
- Eating disorders
- Decreased sun exposure, lower levels of vitamin D
- Not feeling supported mentally and emotionally in school, work, or home
- Lower levels of self-esteem, motivation, and any interest in engaging socially
- Higher levels of social media exposure and engagement

- Feeling alone, depressed, and isolated in one's own struggles
- Not knowing who to turn to
- Loss of a loved one—parent, significant other, friend, relatives, others
- Increase in FOMO (fear of missing out) feelings
- Lack of knowledge and skills for self-care
- Genetic mental health struggles
- Negative thoughts and behaviors
- News events
- Feelings of shame
- Suffering in silence
- Lack of motivation for taking care of mental, physical, emotional, and spiritual health
- Lack of knowledge and skills for building resiliency
- Pressure in someone's personal, educational, or work life
- Physical, mental, and emotional abuse

Mental Health America (MHA) is a national organization dedicated to promoting mental health, prevention services, interventions, early detection of those at risk, and providing care and services. According to data from the *MHA 2022 Mental Health in America* report:

- In 2019, 50 million American adults had a mental illness.
- Suicidal ideation continues to increase every year since 2011, more so in the COVID-19 pandemic.
- The percentages of youth experiencing depression continue to increase.
- More than 2.5 million youth have major depression, and multiracial youth have a greater risk for depression.
- More than 27 million adults in the U.S. do not receive treatment for mental illness.
- More than 60 percent of youth who suffer from severe depression are not receiving treatment.

- Some adults and youth with a mental health illness do not have health insurance or insurance that covers mental health services. In fact, 950,000 youth had private health insurance that did not include mental health coverage.
- Substance abuse is increasing for adults and youth.

On December 7, 2021, the U.S. Department of Health and Human Services shared the following: "U.S. Surgeon General issues advisory on youth mental health crisis further exposed by COVID-19 pandemic." Surgeon General Vivek Murthy announced the urgency of mental health and wellness initiatives:

"Mental health challenges in children, adolescents, and young adults are real and widespread. Even before the pandemic, an alarming number of young people struggled with feelings of helplessness, depression, and thoughts of suicide—and rates have increased over the past decade. The COVID-19 pandemic further altered their experiences at home, school, and in the community, and the effect on their mental health has been devastating. The future well-being of our country depends on how we support and invest in the next generation."[2] My response in reading this was relief in that mental health is finally becoming a priority and there is now more awareness about mental health, but you might be wondering, "Okay, but what can be done about this crisis and how soon?" I know I am.

Higher levels of anxiety, depression, feelings of hopelessness, isolation, loneliness, uncertainty, suicidal ideation, racial and ethnic health disparities, increased drug and alcohol use, and other crises reflect the chaos created by COVID-19. Healthcare professionals, school counselors, teachers, and other health and wellness professionals were pushed beyond their abilities, and many left the workforce. In a

---

[2] Vivek H. Murthy, M.D., M.B.A., Vice Admiral, U.S. Public Health Service, Surgeon General of the United States, "Protecting Youth Mental Health: The U.S. Surgeon General's Advisory," United States Department of Health and Human Services, 2021, www.hhs.gov/sites/default/files/surgeon-general-youth-mental-health-advisory.pdf.

July 2022 article, "The Silver Lining of the Current Mental Health Crisis," Yahoo News shared that the number of people living with a mental illness has dramatically increased, but now people are seeking care to deal with their struggles. Here are some key takeaways:

- More personal and professional struggles resulted in greater demand for mental health services.
- In 2019, one in five American adults were living with a mental illness, and now the number of people suffering with depression has more than tripled (8.5 percent pre-pandemic to 32.8 percent in 2021).
- The World Health Organization reported that anxiety and depression have increased 25 percent internationally.
- People are seeking more support than before the pandemic started.

The next chapter will explore how we ended up in a mental health pandemic, specifically the factors that contributed to the increase in a need for mental healthcare and services, how the world was unprepared for a global pandemic on so many levels, a look at the behaviors that reflect the trauma and chaos inflicted by COVID-19, and how this deadly virus only exacerbated pre-existing mental health challenges.

Buckle up. The year 2020 was a *really* bumpy ride.

CHAPTER 2

The Making of a Mental Health Pandemic

"I thought it was going to be like a really cool break from school for a few weeks, and it turned into two months and then two years, and it's been really annoying, and I hated wearing a mask everywhere."
– Jaden, 14

Mental health affects every aspect of our lives. Our ability to cope day to day while living in a pandemic is no small feat. Individual and societal problem, and stress levels have never been this high, especially for marginalized communities already struggling mentally, emotionally, socially, and financially. Here's a look at how the mental health pandemic came to be.

The Origins of the Mental Health Pandemic

It all began with...

Pre-existing mental, emotional, physical, behavioral conditions
that were kept hidden or not addressed

+

A mental healthcare system that was: broken/already
needing an overhaul, not providing equal access,
not meeting the needs of people struggling

8

+

Lack of resources, emotional and socio-economical support,
lack of knowledge and skills to address mental health
struggles, and social and emotional needs

+

Stigma, gender, and racial inequities,
discrimination of all kinds (ageism,
systematic racism, sexism, biases)

+

**The Disruptor = COVID-19
resulting in a global pandemic
Causing a myriad of societal, socio-economic, mental,
physical, and emotional issues:**
Negative ripple effects of the pandemic
(e.g., millions of people out of work, lockdowns, social distancing,
isolation, depression, anxiety, suicidal ideation, loss, feelings
of hopelessness, substance abuse, mental health programs and
professionals not available to everyone, addiction, physical and
emotional abuse at home, not doing well in school or work, etc.)

+

Increase in personal and professional struggles, especially those
who are teachers, healthcare workers, school
counselors, students, people
with pre-existing struggles of all kinds, etc.

+

Horrific behaviors and news events
(e.g., gun violence, school shootings, millions die
around the globe from COVID-19, long-term effects
of COVID-19, police brutality, racial and ethnic
discrimination and violence, soaring rates of
depression, anxiety, despair, suicide, physical and
emotional abuse, substance abuse, etc.)

+

Further stress and strain on hospitals, healthcare workers, and health and wellness professionals, teachers, and the mental health infrastructure that was already in need of an overhaul within schools, businesses, other organizations, etc.

+

Alcohol and substance abuse
before and/or during COVID-19

+

Lack of preparation to handle the mental, emotional, and physical trauma created by the pandemic

+

Societal fear, anger, polarization on numerous issues

=

Mental Health Pandemic

It's August 8, 2022, and the Johns Hopkins Coronavirus Resource Center (CRC) is reporting the following updates on COVID-19 cases and deaths:

- Total Confirmed Cases, globally—584,450,524
- Total Global Deaths—6,417,782
- U.S. Confirmed Cases—92,112,922
- U.S. Deaths—1,033,556

These numbers alone are enough to keep us up at night, reclusive with our phones, Netflix, and Postmates. By the time I finish writing this book, these numbers will be even higher.

The COVID-19 Timeline

The following COVID-19 timeline is based on information from the Centers for Disease Control and Prevention and the David J. Sencer CDC Museum, as well as a January 9, 2021, article in Newsweek.

com entitled, "A timeline of COVID-19 from discovery to vaccine" by Stephanie Parker, Diana Shishkina, and Betsy Ladyzhets.

Key moments[3]

December 12, 2019

Patients in Wuhan, Hubei Province, China have symptoms of a mysterious upper respiratory illness.

December 30, 2019

Li Wenliang, a Chinese ophthalmologist who worked at Wuhan Central Hospital in Wuhan, China, notifies his colleagues of a new respiratory virus spreading in Wuhan.

December 31, 2019

The World Health Organization China Country Office is notified of numerous cases of pneumonia originating from Huanan Seafood Wholesale Market in Wuhan.

January 2020

Li Wenliang contracts the virus from a patient. First coronavirus death reported in Wuhan is a sixty-one-year-old man who frequently shopped at the Huanan Seafood Wholesale Market.

Cases of the virus spread to Thailand, Japan, and South Korea. An American, who traveled to Wuhan from Washington State, contracts the virus.

---

[3] Stephanie Parker et al. "A Timeline of Covid-19 from Discovery to Vaccine," *Newsweek*, January 9, 2021, https://www.newsweek.com/timeline-covid-19-discovery-vaccine-1559075; Centers for Disease Control and Prevention, "CDC Museum COVID-19 Timeline," accessed February 16, 2023, https://www.cdc.gov/museum/timeline/covid19.html.

January 30, 2020: Thousands of people are infected, and hundreds die

The World Health Organization announces a Public Health Emergency, and travel to and from China is halted by President Donald Trump.

February 7, 2020

Li Wenliang dies from the virus.

February 11, 2020: The virus is named COVID-19

The World Health Organization names the disease spread by the novel coronavirus: COVID-19.

February 2020

I exit a local library in Orange County, California, and see a small shrine dedicated to the late Li Wenliang. I begin to see more and more stories of COVID-19 in the news.

March 2020

Over 100,000 cases worldwide. The WHO declares COVID-19 as a global pandemic. Mid-March, the U.S. begins to shut down schools, businesses, bars, and restaurants to prevent the spread of COVID-19.

Over 3.3. million people file for unemployment.

The Coronavirus Aid, Relief, and Economic Security Act (CARES Act) is a $2.2 trillion economic stimulus bill passed by the 116th U.S. Congress, signed into law by President Donald Trump.

U.S. residents who were eligible began receiving $1,200 stimulus payments and an increase in unemployment benefits.

April 2020

Over 1 million COVID-19 cases. Protests over the stay-at-home orders.

July 2020

The U.S. has over 4 million cases and over 145,000 deaths.

August 26, 2020

The Abbott Diagnostics antigen test is approved.

November 4, 2020

The U.S. has over 100,000 cases in a day.

December 2, 2020

U.S. hospitals caring for record number of COVID-19 patients—over 100,000.

December 2020

The U.S. Food and Drug Administration gives emergency authorization to Moderna and Pfizer vaccinations.

Our Outdated, Dysfunctional Mental Healthcare System

I want to set the stage for how we got to where we are in our current mental health pandemic. I am by no means a mental health professional, and I don't pretend to be one. I do, however speak to people of all ages about their personal struggles, mental health challenges, support systems or lack thereof, and personal journeys into trying to make sense out of the chaos we are living in. Some conversations in this book were supposed to last thirty minutes. Sometimes, we spoke for two hours. Those two hours were often the highlight of my day. I felt honored and connected to a new human I had just met. We both needed space to share, vent, and connect in a time of disconnect, and sometimes, it was also nice to have reassurance that the work I am doing really matters and makes a difference.

To explain the state of our current mental health pandemic and how we got here, I am going to use the analogy of a house. Think of our U.S. mental healthcare system as a house that has been around a LONG time. Let's say the house is a home built in the 1800s with old rickety floors and wood beams; it's a mess. The house hasn't been inspected and updated at all; there's probably decay, mold, termites, lead paint, asbestos, and a whole bunch of other unsafe issues. It's just an old house that no one tended to. People have come in from time to time and thrown a few coats of paint on, new curtains, rugs, and new furniture, but at its core, it's still an old, neglected house.

The house *really* needs an update. All the other homes in the neighborhood now had high-speed internet and smart technology, but this house still had rotary phones (some of you won't know what those are! LOL) and not enough people to take care of the house. One day, the owners started paying more attention to the house, and they had people come in to tackle a huge list of upgrades and repairs. Without updating the infrastructure of the house, they thought they would just make some cosmetic repairs and promote it as an Airbnb.

The problem was the house had never been upgraded, and there was so much to do. People didn't communicate well and think about the priorities and what people staying at the house would need and want. The owners hired clueless people to make upgrades, and the repair people were overwhelmed because there was a tight timeframe to do everything. No one was on the same page, and it wasn't clear what the long-term plan for the house would be. There were not enough time and resources to do everything, and the real problems with the house were not even addressed (e.g., slab leaks, rotting floors).

The house was then promoted in a glitzy brand marketing campaign, and someone rented it out. Little did the renters know, they would not be getting what they paid for. The cost of upgrades and repairs was expensive, and the people who owned the house couldn't afford to do it all. To top it off, the people working on the house weren't compensated enough, often mistreated, disrespected, and couldn't handle all the problems that resulted from neglect and apathy. They quit out of frustration and mistreatment; many left to do something else and not even in the field they were skilled in.

A massive storm was brewing, and the news outlets warned everyone that this one was going to be a doozy of a storm. When the heavy rain and high-speed winds hit the house, the roof split in two, and the neglected home was no match for the chaos and strength of the storm. The owners were out of touch (literally and figuratively) on vacation; they didn't consider that the storm would devastate the home and the people living in it. When they did return, they sought the original repair crew to fix things, but they were nowhere to be found; the house was in disrepair, and no one had a clue how to make the repairs and upgrades.

I think you get the idea. The house represents the mental healthcare system that has long been neglected. No one prioritized its care and updating. Now, we live in a time when the pandemic storm has ripped the roof off of our lives and revealed a healthcare system that needed an overhaul yesterday. Policymakers, educators, businesses, and other stakeholders must agree on the basic structure and rebuild, so we can provide the proper training and education and get the skilled and talented and resources needed to address the needs of those struggling socially, emotionally, and mentally. We must also value those who work in education, healthcare, and other essential positions who sacrifice their own safety and well-being because they are passionate and driven to make a difference.

Positive psychologist Sonja Lyubomirsky, author of *The How of Happiness* published in 2007, developed the Subjective Happiness

Scale, which measures our subjective happiness. Lyubomirsky shares that happiness is affected by three things: life's circumstances, genetics, and the choices we make.

With Lyubomirsky's research in mind, I considered how happiness was affected during the pandemic. Our happiness levels plummeted, and not surprisingly. Happiness and our ability to stay positive and optimistic has been affected by:

1. Life circumstances not in our control—We had no control over this life-changing disruptor, COVID-19, resulting in lockdowns, working from home, job loss, social isolation, and so many other scenarios.
2. Genetics—If we were pre-disposed to depression, anxiety, substance abuse, manic depression, bipolar disorder, and other mental health issues, we went deeper into a rabbit hole or maybe experienced a darker side to ourselves because of trauma, either recent or in childhood.
3. Our choices—When faced with COVID-19 and everything that happened because of the virus, we might have experienced negative thoughts and behaviors, which could be detrimental to our minds, bodies, emotions, and relationships. Drugs, alcohol, vaping, tech addiction, anti-social behavior, and other negative behaviors help people numb out. These negative choices dramatically affect us mental, physical, and emotionally.

June 17, 2022

The World Health Organization published an urgent report to overhaul our mental healthcare system and mental health initiatives. "Report urges mental health decision makers and advocates to step up commitment and action to change attitudes, actions and approaches to mental health, its determinants and mental health care." The 2022 scientific report by the WHO found that the COVID-19 pandemic caused a 25 percent global increase in anxiety and depression. Some of the major factors contributing to this are social isolation, loneliness, fear of getting sick and dying, losing loved ones, grief, lack of sufficient mental healthcare services, and financial issues.[4]

No one has been immune to the effects of the COVID-19 pandemic. Our world has been hit by a tidal wave of disappointment, personal, professional, and financial chaos and loss, mental health struggles, and unexpected life changing circumstances that no one could have planned for. I set out to explore how people experienced the pandemic, what we can learn from these challenging times, and how we can become better humans, because the fact is—we need to. We must reconnect with ourselves and prioritize mental, physical, and emotional health as a society while also becoming more compassionate, empathetic individuals.

Before the pandemic began, the topic of mental health had never been this prevalent in the media. From online news, TV reports, and social media posts, people of all ages began sharing their personal stories and struggles, necessitating a societal mindset and structural overhaul. The following quote from *New York Times* columnist Jessica Grose captures just how stressed and maxed out mothers felt in 2021: "It's not just the working from home, the record unemployment, or the remote schooling. The coronavirus pandemic has unleashed a mental health crisis, too. This is a primal scream."

The pandemic had such a traumatic impact on mothers that the *New York Times* created an eighteen-page section in The Primal Scream Series entitled, "America's Mothers are in Crisis. Is anyone listening to them?"[5] The groundbreaking section included research findings,

---

4   World Health Organization, "WHO highlights urgent need to transform mental health and mental health care," June 17, 2022, https://www.who.int/news/item/17-06-2022-who-highlights-urgent-need-to-transform-mental-health-and-mental-health-care.

5   Jessica Grose, "America's Mothers Are In Crisis: Is anyone listening to them?" *The New York Times*, February 4, 2021, www.nytimes.com/2021/02/04/parenting/working-moms-mental-health-coronavirus.html.

evidence of racial disparities, and quotes of trauma, exhaustion, hope, perseverance, and chaos. Surveys on race and health revealed Black and Hispanic women without partners experienced life-changing negative impacts from the pandemic. Mothers more so than fathers experienced job loss, physiological issues, and trouble sleeping. The Center for WorkLife Law reported a 700 percent increase in calls from working parents to their crisis hotline.

The next chapter will look at the pandemic events that fueled the mental health pandemic, tragic news that shaped our collective trauma nationally and internationally, a timeline of U.S. events that became embedded in our minds and news feeds, and a look at how the media reflected a domino effect of fallout from the pandemic—the ongoing emotional and mental turmoil ignited by COVID-19.

CHAPTER 3

Fueling the Mental Health Pandemic

"I think that the younger generation has been a lot more exposed and globally aware of the stuff that's been going on, which I think is good, but also there is that anxiousness that comes from that. You know about the things that are going on halfway across the world and feel weird and anxious that it would happen to you. Ukrainian people are struggling, and they have to move out of their homes. There's a lot of anxiety. Knowing that's happening across the world, makes you feel uncomfortable and anxious in school or whatever you're doing."
—Sriya Chilla, [17]

March 2022 marked two years since the World Health Organization declared that COVID-19 was a global pandemic. The American Psychological Association, in partnership with The Harris Poll, conducted a Stress in America™ survey in February 2022 and then in early March 2022. The top sources of stress noted by participants in the survey include:

- 87 percent—Increase in prices due to inflation
- 81 percent—Issues with the supply chain
- 81 percent—Global uncertainty
- 80 percent—Concerns about Russia retaliating

- 80 percent—Russia's invasion of Ukraine

The study also revealed that watching the war in Ukraine has caused an increase in fear. Sixty-nine percent of those surveyed worry the war will result in a nuclear war. Eighty-seven percent of adults feel that there has been one crisis after the next over the past two years, and seventy-three percent are overwhelmed by what is happening in the world. Concerns about money, the economy and housing continue to be a significant source of stress for ages eighteen to forty-three. Latino adults had the most concerns about money, the economy, and housing, followed by Black adults, White adults, and Asian adults.[6]

The mental health pandemic is being fueled by COVID-19, specifically factors resulting from the disruption of life as we knew it, the ripple effects of the pandemic, and national and global news events, such as the war in Ukraine. Pre-existing mental health issues have been exacerbated by life in a pandemic. Many people with substance abuse issues are more prone to an increase in addiction, and those who were struggling financially, emotionally, or for other reasons had an even more difficult life during the onset of COVID-19. In a 2022 WHO report, findings reveal that younger people and women have been affected tremendously. They are more prone to self-harm and suicidal thoughts, especially if they have pre-existing mental illnesses.

Events that Shaped our Collective Trauma

Collective trauma is an emotional response to a fearful life event that can threaten your life and bring about feelings of helplessness.

When COVID-19 spread, your reality was turned upside down. You most likely experienced a traumatic response to the ripple effects

---

[6]   American Psychological Association, "Stress in America," 2022, https://www.apa.org/news/press/releases/stress/2022/march-2022-survival-mode

of the pandemic, and you were not alone. Millions felt the disruption and uncertainty, the stress, and anxiety of collective trauma. How could you not? Millions of people died from COVID-19, and rates of anxiety, trauma, depression, suicidal thoughts, and suicide soared. The need for psychological counseling outweighed the availability of mental health professionals. Drug use increased, as did vaping, alcohol consumption, binge watching, social media usage, and incidents of drug addiction and overdose. Fear, anxiety, depression, hopelessness, and trauma associated with COVID-19 and national and international news events, added to the long list of issues associated with the mental health pandemic, such as:

- Gun violence
- School shootings
- War in Ukraine
- Loss of connection
- Constraints on people's lives
- Loneliness
- Social isolation
- Fear of getting sick and dying
- Loss of a loved one
- Fear of losing a job
- Losing a job
- Alcohol and substance abuse
- Financial and emotional stress due to job loss or changes at work
- Overturning of Roe v. Wade
- Schools, administrators, and policies not meeting the mental and emotional needs of students, teachers, and staff
- Healthcare workers burning out from stress and trauma
- Teachers leaving their field because of stress, trauma, being overworked, an increase in workload, underappreciated, and undercompensated

- Businesses not meeting the mental and emotional needs of employees
- Exhaustion and hopelessness from a life affected by COVID-19

Here are some top news events that were fueled by the mental health pandemic from 2020 to present:

Hate Crimes. Hate crimes against marginalized groups—based on race, religion, cultures, gender, socio-economic status, and age—increased.

The Murder of George Floyd. Police brutality before and during the pandemic was on the rise, and then there was the horrific murder of George Floyd in 2020 in front of many witnesses. Floyd, a forty-six-year-old Black man, was murdered by Derek Chauvin, a forty-four-year-old White police officer in Minneapolis, while many people, including other police officers, watched. This horrific incident became a catalyst for nationwide protests against police brutality.

The Capitol Riots. In 2021, after U.S. President Donald Trump's defeat in the 2020 presidential election, a mob of Trump supporters attacked the Capitol building in Washington, D.C. They violently stormed the building, scaling walls, breaking windows, vandalizing, looting, and terrorizing staff inside the building. Their goal was to keep Trump in power as president and disrupt the counting of the electoral votes that would secure the presidential win of President-elect Joe Biden.

The Overturning of Roe v. Wade. This decision impacts the mental and emotional health of young girls through adulthood. The announcement sent shockwaves throughout the nation.

The rise of political polarization in the U.S. has been on full display for decades, but the past few years feel like a bigger showcase of negativity for all the world to see. Political parties disagree on a myriad of issues, enhanced by societal disagreement, conflict, distrust, and media coverage. Hostility rears its ugly head on social media, news talk radio, and TV, and aggressive behaviors throughout society reflect the inability of people to agree, disagree, and have healthy exchanges while acting civilized. Disagreement with the common goal of betterment can be a way to fuel positive change. Unfortunately, not everyone is there yet.

2022 shootings

- Ten people died from a racially motivated shooting at Tops Supermarket in Buffalo, N.Y.
- A school shooting at an elementary school in Uvalde, Texas, killed nineteen children and two adults.
- NPR Reporter Jaclyn Diaz reported that Uvalde is the twenty-seventh school shooting this year.[7]
- At a Fourth of July parade in Highland Park, Illinois, seven died while over thirty were injured when a gunman started shooting.
- According to the Gun Violence Archive, there have been at least 309 mass shootings as of July 4, 2022. Gun violence increased during the pandemic.

COVID-19 and mental health made headlines. The news was a constant reflection of our world in crisis:

- There was a rise in substance abuse due to COVID-19 stress and anxiety.
- School shootings created an aftermath of fear, stress, and anxiety.
- COVID-19 impacted racial and ethnic groups differently.

---

[7] Jaclyn Diaz, "27 school shootings have taken place so far this year," *NPR*, May 25, 2022, https://www.npr.org/2022/05/24/1101050970/2022-school-shootings-so-far.

- The virus took a serious toll on the mental health of children.
- Coronavirus affected the mental health of millennials and Generation Z.
- Over 170,000 children lost parents or caregivers to COVID-19.
- Crime rates increased, as did racism—e.g., hate crimes against Asian American and Pacific Islander communities rose during the pandemic.
- Before the pandemic, teens were experiencing a mental health crisis:
  - COVID-19 caused an increase in anxiety and depression globally
  - Alcohol-related deaths increased during the COVID-19 pandemic
- The mental health of Generation Z declined during the pandemic.
- More people sought help for mental health issues and illnesses.
- Suicidal thoughts and self-harm increased during the pandemic for LGBTQ youth.
- Racial and ethnic disparities impacted mental health.
- Teen mental health declined due to loss of income, parental stress, and emotional abuse.
- The pandemic revealed past and present trauma for all ages.
- Gun violence and COVID-19 strained the U.S. healthcare system. The U.S. Surgeon General warned of a severe shortage of healthcare workers due to burnout.
- In 2022, a CNN/Kaiser Family Foundation research study found that 90 percent of adults said there is a mental health crisis.

When our world went into lockdown in March 2020, you (like many other people did) might have thought the virus would last a few weeks or a couple of months. No one expected our world would unravel, infiltrating lives with one crisis after the next, and taking a toll on millions of people. The pandemic disrupted daily routines and expectations, from school and work to relationships, social gatherings, and limiting any type of physical interaction. Children of all ages and young adults missed out on the memories and milestones of school and college life that their parents experienced growing up. You might have been one of the millions of college students who had to move back home, spending the first few years of college online, changing plans about what and where to study, choosing a different career/life path in the COVID-19 economy, and where to live now that COVID-19 had disrupted your life. Parents who were paying for college tuition soon had their young adult restricted to remote learning with no college life for the same price tag. Disappointment, stress, depression, anxiety, relationship problems, and more became more prevalent in lockdown.

Now in 2022, life for school-aged children means growing up practicing active-shooter drills in preparation for future gun violence. Just the thought of this makes me anxious and scared for children who have to even consider this frightening scenario, but sadly, this is the world we live in now. Issues that matter to students and parents now include gun control and mental health initiatives. Some people even want school personnel to carry weapons. A little later on, Octavio Hernandez, a Florida teacher featured in the *New York Times*, will share his views on teachers carrying guns.

All the feels—and not the good ones…

During the COVID-19 pandemic, you might have experienced one or more of the following psychological and physiological reactions. Which ones apply to you?

- Fear
- Anxiety
- Depression

- Suicidal thoughts or actions
- Self-harm
- Isolation
- Hopelessness
- Inability to concentrate
- Loss of appetite
- Uncontrollable worrying
- Panic attacks
- Low interest in doing things you normally enjoy
- Anti-social behavior
- Nightmares
- Insomnia
- Hopelessness
- Headaches and body aches
- Stomach issues
- Negative self-soothing actions
- Increased use of drugs, alcohol, or other numbing out activities
- Anger
- Uncontrollable worry
- Despair
- Trauma, past or present

With the advancements of technology came great havoc, from the lure and addiction of our cell phones to the negative effects of overusing the technology, compromising our relationships and our inabilities to be present and mindful when we are in-person. Adding to the turmoil is the deep political divide in our country and the long overdue conversations about discrimination against people based on their race, ethnicity, gender, religion, sexual orientation, disability or illness, age, socioeconomic status, and political views. You might have experienced discrimination if you are Latino, Indigenous, Asian, BIPOC, LGBTQIA, or part of another marginalized community. It took a pandemic to shake up the world and make people see that toxic behavior is detrimental and has to stop. I can't help but think of Grammy award–winning artist Lizzo and the title of her viral song, "About Damn Time."

You are hooked to your electronic devices like pacifiers and soothers in awkward social situations, and I admit, so am I. There is a constant need to check our phones to see who called, texted, and responded to social media posts. Each time there is a notification, our brains release dopamine. As this happens, we check our phones even more for that rush of dopamine. App developers have intentionally lured us away from being present in the moment. These handheld devices have impacted lives beyond awareness. The lure of technology is mind numbing, more so during the pandemic. You might be unaware of how being on your phone makes the other person sitting across from you feel; they just want to be heard and seen and know that you are fully present—not half listening while texting and checking your phone. Like a lot of people, you might be tethered to your phone but feel the loneliest you have ever felt. Being on your phone feels comforting, and you can't go without checking it throughout the day; this is the sad state of humanity. I am just as guilty of this addictive behavior. I need to take a trip someday, shut my phone off, and soak in my surroundings. We'll see how long I can last.

For many of us, being in person after a long time of social isolation can be awkward. You might feel more comfortable saying what is on your mind through technology. Addiction to social media and the need to have more likes and follows has exploded. The irony is that someone can have thousands and even millions of likes on a video they created but very few followers. To me, that seems like millions of people saying hello and liking your cool new sneakers, but you really only have five friends, and what does that translate into anyway? We focus so much on gaining followers and connections, thinking that those numbers are our gateways into opportunities and popularity. Oftentimes, however, they are not; it's just like one big popularity contest that makes us feel good when we know thousands of people liked something we posted.

Social media is not even an accurate view of reality most of the time. Many creators struggle with their own personal demons, insecurities, and challenges. As a creator, you focus on who liked your last post, what others are saying about all the hard work you put into those TikTok videos and Instagram reels and stories. Unread texts or texts read and not responded to are seriously upsetting. The feeling of rejection, missing out, and dissatisfaction with your life and making comparisons, with a heavy dose of "not being good enough," fills our thoughts and shifts our moods. The truth is—this is all toxic and detrimental to our thoughts, feelings, behaviors, and relationships of all kinds, including our relationships with ourselves.

If Swedish climate activist Greta Thunberg could inspire millions of people to walk out of school for climate change, why is our society not as passionate about mental health? In 2018, when she was fifteen, Thunberg began protesting outside of the Swedish Parliament. She challenged world leaders to take a stand on climate change and initiated the first-ever school strike to raise awareness about the issue. She inspired millions of people of all ages to lead their own climate change strikes throughout the world. She tuned out the brutal negativity of opponents, with former President Donald Trump and other critics even remarking on the fact that she has Asperger's syndrome. We need more Gretas in the world. I don't know about you, but I would be the first in line to walk out for mental health.

Stress, trauma, anxiety, and other negative life events fueled the mental health pandemic. How are *YOU* doing through all of this? Pandemic events—unconscionable deaths, violence, soaring rates of COVID-19, coronavirus variants, life disruptions, mask mandates, social isolation, loneliness, and horrific news stories—are now part of our "new normal." I really don't like that phrase. Our old normal wasn't so normal, just our life on autopilot. We focused on ourselves, our achievements, status, materialism, the size of our paychecks, titles that really mean nothing, and living in a fast-paced world that never paused to gain any introspection of what was broken and needed repair—all while not paying attention to the people around us who were suffering all along.

Let's check in and see how you fared. *Check all that apply to you*:

- ☐ Disappointment because your plans were no longer a reality
- ☐ Loneliness and social isolation
- ☐ Stress, anxiety, depression suicidal thoughts/behaviors fueled by COVID-19
- ☐ Substance abuse
- ☐ Getting COVID-19 and experiencing long-term effects that hinder your life
- ☐ Stress of debt
- ☐ Food insecurity
- ☐ Disruption of your home life (e.g., having to move, losing your house, etc.)
- ☐ Not being able to see family and friends
- ☐ Getting separated or divorced
- ☐ Racial and ethnic disparities
- ☐ Discrimination against Asians, BIPOC, LGBTQ, multiracial LGBTQ couples, etc.
- ☐ Increased political polarization
- ☐ Violence, abuse
- ☐ Losing a loved one or fur baby
- ☐ Losing a loved one and not being able to see them before they passed away
- ☐ Cancelled plans—travel, milestones, etc.
- ☐ Loss of several people—friends, family, partner, etc.
- ☐ Loss of opportunities—jobs, internships, etc.
- ☐ Quitting your job
- ☐ Cancelled milestones
- ☐ Financial loss
- ☐ Disruption of your living situation

- Not having enough food to eat
- Not knowing where you will live
- Being diagnosed with COVID-19 and living in fear and anxiety
- Being diagnosed with something else
- Not being able to live the life you expected (e.g., go to college and experience what your parents did)
- Pre-pandemic mental health struggles now worsening
- Social isolation affecting all ages
- The impact of missed milestones on tweens, teens, and beyond

If you are a young adult, you might have had to move back home, make decisions about what to study, what your career/life path looks like now in the COVID economy, and where to live now that the virus hijacked your plans. The pandemic shook up your life, from school and work to relationships, social gatherings, and connecting with others. You missed out on the memories and milestones of school and college life that your parents experienced growing up. No one could really grasp what it felt like to sit in your shoes and how your life felt like an uphill battle.

If you were confined to your bedroom and school was online, you might have struggled to learn. Not everyone was equipped to learn online, too; maybe your internet connection was not fast enough or you didn't have a computer or laptop you can use to work remotely. Where, then, did that leave those who had to face this new world of remote learning? A Pew Research study in May 2020 showed that many young adults lost internships and jobs; this affected their mental and emotional health, increasing stress and anxiety levels. Having seen their Gen X parents struggle in the recession, Generation Z was already focused pre-pandemic on making smart financial decisions and choosing careers that paid well. If you graduated and persevered through this pandemic, your resilience and adaptability shined bright, and this speaks volumes about your ability to pivot and adapt in times of change and unpredictability.

In the next chapter, you will hear from several young adults, mostly Generation Z and a few younger millennials, who share what their life was like growing up in a pandemic, the challenges they faced before and during COVID-19, and their visions for how we can find our way out of the mental health pandemic. I have always admired these youth leaders, their insights into change, and how they managed through these emotionally challenging times.

CHAPTER 4

Youth Leaders in Mental Health and Wellness

"I think one thing that teachers and staff at school have to keep in mind is that academics follow mental health."
—*Sriya Chilla, UCLA freshman*

Today's children, teens, and young adults have been significantly impacted by COVID-19. They struggled mentally, emotionally, financially, physically, academically, and socially. Yes, millions of students could learn online, but what about others who could not afford a computer, a therapist, food on their table, and other necessities? Some depended on their schools for meals, emotional support, and counseling. There was very little preparation for the new remote reality in March 2020, and today's youth did not fare well.

There is no question that Gen Z and Millennials have had a rough time growing up in a pandemic. They see the impact of the pandemic, experiencing hardships no one would have imagined; it's been nothing short of a shit show filled with one curveball after another. No wonder they have had a hard time managing everyday life with such an enormous ripple effect of issues to process. If you fit into the Gen Z or millennial demographic, you probably experienced stress, depression, anxiety, suicidal thoughts, and trauma, even before the pandemic. Every new variant caused more negative news and an increase in mental, emotional, and economic duress. With the news instantly at your fingertips, how can anyone not be compassionate with the life you are faced with every day? Add the mass shootings to the mix, the increase in suicide rates, depression and opioid crisis, and the stress of social media comparisons and distortions of reality, and the pandemic has only made matters worse.

No matter how old you are, you most likely lost a friend, family member, teacher, internship, job, or missed numerous rites of passage. One thing that has remained is your outspoken beliefs about mental health, humanitarian efforts, climate issues, social and civic engagements, racism, discrimination, gender identity, and equality. You have awakened the world to issues that were long suppressed, dismissed, and overlooked. You know you have inherited societal problems that need solutions now, not just conversation.

In 2020, my then eighteen-year-old daughter asked me to go to a peaceful protest for the Black Lives Matter movement and against the horrifying deaths of George Floyd, Breonna Taylor, and numerous other Black men and woman who died at the hands of police. As I watched her finish making a large poster with the names of lives lost to police brutality, I knew this was an opportunity for me to learn and expand my viewpoint. We donned our masks and drove to the event and stood with hundreds of people of all ages with a desire to protest senseless racial atrocities and seek out societal change. The moment of silence and the emotionally moving speeches are a memory I will never forget. Attending this event connected me even more with my daughter, and to the issues at hand. Most importantly, as a White woman, I was reminded to check my White privilege.

In a 2016 article by Mehak Anwar on Bustle.com, she reminds us:

"There are a variety of reasons it's important to check your white privilege if you're a white or white-presenting person, but the number one reason it's crucial to do so is to not become or remain complicit in a racist system that values the lives and experiences of one group over another based on something so arbitrary."

At the protest, my daughter and I were drawn to the tear-filled voices of Generation Z speaking to the crowd. This was a moment to stand outside of my own reality, gain greater perspective on racial discrimination and how discrimination is influenced by appearance, socioeconomic status, ethnicity, gender identification, level of education, age, religion, sexual identity, and ability. The protest shifted my awareness of how I see the world and how we all play a role in bringing about meaningful, societal change that connects us instead of causing further division.

According to a February 14, 2021 article by The Annie E. Casey Foundation, entitled "Social issues That Matter to Generation Z," growing up with technology has meant that "Gen Zers have been able to connect to faraway cultures, issues and news earlier and more often than any generation before them. As a result, Generation Z members tend to be more open-minded, liberal-leaning and actively engaged in advocating for the fair and equal treatment of others."[8] I admire how this generation is tuned into issues that matter deeply, especially when their future is filled with problems inherited from past generations (i.e., systemic racism, environmental issues causing health problems—cancer, economic instability).

For students with pre-existing struggles in school (mentally, socially, or academically), the world of online learning created additional challenges, such as an increase in depression. Conversely speaking, perhaps you thrived from being remote and limiting your social anxiety. You might have found yourself in an academic spiral, turned your computer camera off during class, and completely disengaged from your teachers, classmates, and subject matter. At a time when you looked forward to connecting with your classmates and attending school events, your life was shattered, so who could blame you for feeling disinterested and disconnected? What was there to look forward to if you knew your school events were cancelled,

[8]   The Annie E. Casey Foundation, "Social Issues That Matter to Generation Z," February 14, 2021,

and graduation was online? For parents, your teen or young adult might have spent more time retreating to their room to sleep and disconnect from you and the world—physically and emotionally. Once we realized the pandemic was here to stay, there were only so many game nights and Zoom family gatherings you could handle. There would never be another generation that would go through the magnitude of chaos caused by a pandemic. And if there ever was, they would learn a lot from today's young adults, who have a lot to say about what matters most right now.

Meet Sriya Chilla

UCLA freshman—Fall 2022
Chair of the Youth Advisory Board at the
California Coalition for Youth (CCY)
Co-Chair of the Community Affairs Committee at the California
Mental Health Advocates for Youth and Children (CMHACY)
Crisis Counselor at the California Youth Crisis Line (CYCL)

"If you're not doing well mentally, even if you're sitting in class and listening or watching the teacher lecture, are you really taking in that information?

Are you going to remember it at the end of the day or at the end of the week?

Are you going to test well? So, academics always follow mental health, and I think it's important to address those mental health needs."

—Sriya Chilla

Sriya is a student at University of California Los Angeles (UCLA) majoring in psychobiology. She always wanted to be a psychiatrist and works as a crisis counselor at the California Youth crisis line.

Here is our conversation about mental health, her desire to help those who are struggling, and her ideas for societal change.

Sriya Chilla (SC): I love talking to people and I love understanding mental illness and making the public policy change that needs to happen. Mentally ill people need to have the support they need in their community and throughout the state and get the care they need.

Janeane Bernstein (JB): According to the website, CMHACY advances the social emotional and behavioral well-being of children and families and promotes inclusion racial equity and social justice for all through convening education and advocacy. Tell me how you got involved in this organization.

SC: I participated in my first conference May 2021, and I was on the youth board panel.

JB: Has this helped you in a lot of ways during the pandemic?

SC: I think [it helps] being able to actually take action toward what I'm seeing in school. I make friends every day because the pandemic has given me more strength. I've been able to refer other youth to leadership positions around mental health so that they can also speak their truth and make their voice heard.

JB: What do you think about the struggles that students have? We were in a mental health crisis, and now we're in a mental health pandemic.

SC: I think the pandemic just exasperated all of the problems that we've already seen because of that lack of social connection and face to face connection and relationships. Feeling alone with your problems is ten times worse than being with your problems around other people and being able to talk to other people. What I've seen a lot coming back to school is a lot of social apathy and a loss of connectedness that I think we use to feel a lot more competitiveness with each other, more judgment, rather than acceptance that we should be having because we've all been through the pandemic, and you've all faced the same struggles.

JB: Do you see people who have changed a lot? Maybe some of your peers don't want to socialize. They're staying home more. They're not as outgoing as they used to be.

SC: Yeah, I think I've seen a lot of that. I'm a senior right now in high school, and we're done with college apps. We're deciding on which college we're going to and deciding on our future essentially, but a lot of people are still afraid of COVID and that's an understandable fear. I've also seen a lot of people that just stay home because they don't want to interact with others. They'd rather just stay in their room playing video games or just doing something with screen time, rather than connecting in person, which we're more able to do now that the lockdowns are done.

JB: At first, people had to be on Zoom and weren't happy about it; they were depressed about it, and then got used to it. Now, it's hard to go back to being in person.

SC: Yeah, I think especially because we're growing socially, having that like, weird halt of two years when we had to learn how to be online halted our social skills in person. I definitely think that people would rather interact online now than in person. Just because of comfortability with being online for the past few years. But that's not something that's going to stay for the rest of our lives. These are social skills in person or something that we do have to learn. We do have to get out and meet each other in person.

JB: Before the pandemic, did you have friends who were struggling with their mental health?

SC: Oh, yeah, for sure. I come from a really competitive high school in San Diego, and we definitely have a lot of that like not feeling enough. We've had a bunch of stuff where people get kicked out of friend groups because they're not taking enough APs or taking up challenging courses. That definitely impacts your own self-worth and how you see yourself. So yeah, we definitely had a lot of mental health problems before the pandemic.

JB: Did you feel like it was hard for you to be successful academically during the pandemic?

SC: Yeah, I just felt a lack of motivation because for me, the fun of school was learning and being with others and growing together. So that was definitely something that I've talked to a lot of my friends about. We didn't really feel like going to class. We didn't feel like it also because all of the social and political things that were going on during that time period. We felt that school was useless when you compare it to the big, larger scope of things, like Black Lives Matter, protests, and all of this other stuff that just felt more important and more urgent than school.

JB: Do you spend a lot of time on your phone, looking at news feeds? I would if I was your age. Is that where you get all your news? If so, do you feel anxious watching that stuff?

SC: Yeah, I'm guilty of that. And I think it permeates into social media, which again, has a good and bad side. Even if you just take a break and go on social media and talk to your friends, something newsworthy will pop up on your feed, and that again creates those feelings of anxiety.

JB: I agree, and I've been hearing a lot of people say there is the good and the bad. When Greta Thunberg left her country and inspired millions of students to protest climate change and leave school, I thought that was incredibly powerful.

SC: Yeah, for sure. Remember the school shooting in Florida? When that happened, our generation took to social media to advocate for the gun violence policy changes that we wanted to see. So, it definitely does have a positive impact.

JB: I really admire your generation because you're very passionate about issues that matter to you and to your future that we should have been paying attention to, and we weren't.

SC: I admire my generation, too. I think this is the change that we need to see in the world. And I think our generation is taking the first step toward that, and hopefully other generations will also follow.

I shared with Sriya that I have noticed her generation seems comfortable saying "I need a mental health day" or "I'm taking care of my mental health." Those phrases are very common among them, whereas someone older might not feel as comfortable saying it because it was not something that was accepted and admired during their time. Here's what she had to say:

SC: I was just talking to a teacher about this like a week ago. She said that even just walking around the classroom and stuff, she can see people sitting at table groups—strangers, not friends—[and hear them] talk to each other about how they're feeling. [They would say] things like, "Oh yeah, yesterday I stayed up all night because I had this assignment to finish with this essay or whatever it is. And I'm feeling kind of sad about it, anxious about my grade or feeling tired. I really don't feel like working today." We're much more open with sharing our thoughts and feelings. And I think that's good. It's definitely an amazing thing that we've kind of developed, but it needs to be followed up and appreciated by staff at school.

JB: Teachers have goals and deadlines and academic procedures they have to focus on, but do you feel that there needs to be better policies in place so mental health can take priority in schools?

SC: Definitely. I think one thing that teachers and staff at school have to keep in mind is that academics follow mental health. If you're not doing mentally well, even if you're sitting in class and listening or like watching the teacher lecture, are you really taking in that information? Are you going to remember it at the end of the day or at the end of the week? Are you going to test well? Academics always follow mental health, and I think it's important to address those mental health needs.

Sriya took a moment to reflect on life before the pandemic and her memory of a traumatic community event. Her teacher made sure to prioritize students' feelings and emotions that day.

SC: I remember before the pandemic, I think it was in tenth grade, something traumatic happened in my community, and one of my teachers just took the day to address the situation. She pushed back all of the scheduling, all of the things we had to talk about what we felt about the situation and what we're feeling with stress and anxiety, and just the political events that were surrounding us. I think that was a really open discussion where we could let her know what we were feeling. She could let us know what she was feeling.

And we could let each other know what we were feeling, so we didn't feel alone. I see teachers taking that step forward, but I think, policy-wise, more needs to be implemented in schools. What I'm advocating for currently is peer-to-peer programs where students can support other students. We know our struggles the most. We live in the same era. We understand what one another are going through.

JB: I love that you said that because I've been saying that in the work I do. I feel that adults can't assume "*this* is what you need," because you're really the customer. It's about what *you* need, and I believe that if there are more peer-to-peer programs and initiatives for you to connect to, then it takes the pressure off of teachers and counselors, who already feel overwhelmed. And yes, you can go to that counselor if something is really bad, but maybe you participate in peer-to-peer initiatives to help you resolve your struggles. Your peers might empathize with what you're going through, and you can work through something together.

SC: And being able to open the conversation with other students and make them comfortable sharing their mental health needs—that kind of bridges the gap between mental health professionals, school psychologists, and the peers because if there's something really serious going on, the peer counselor feels overwhelmed with or incapable of handling for any reason, or a crisis is happening, they can refer that student over to the school psychologist, physically walking them to the school psychologist office, and establishing that connection. Because right now, I know from my personal experience and my friends' experiences, we're not using the mental health professionals who are on campus. And so that's the best way to bridge that gap.

JB: I'm hearing that too. Students are not going to mental health professionals within the school. They just don't feel that they're heard, or they don't feel comfortable going to that person. So, they don't go.

SC: Yeah. I think it's that generational gap where how can you expect someone who's maybe thirty-four years old to understand what it's like to be seventeen in this new era. No offense, but they were in high school long ago.

JB: Right. And you've missed milestones in the pandemic, and you've gone through certain things. No one can really understand unless they're part of your generation. I would love to see more adults be receptive to peer-to-peer initiatives, because I believe that holds a lot of power.

SC: And it starts with each county because we know that in California each county is so different from the next. It starts with county leaders starting an initiative to make this a thing in all schools. Our goal is to get this established in all California high schools. And so having the counties on board is really important for us to accomplish that goal. And then we work our way up to the state. There's a couple of bills that are going through the Assembly and Senate right now that give funding to those that structure peer-to-peer (initiatives). We're looking into that right now.

The organization supports a lot of different mental health initiatives. And one of the ones that I had another youth board member working on is peer-to-peer. We're also working with a lot of other people who used to be on the board; they are helping us with finding the funding that's coming down from Governor Newsom and the state to fund peer-to-peer programs as a whole structure that could actually be existing on campus. The organization just finished a conference. Our theme was not business as usual but conversation to action. We focused a lot on the action part of policy because usually we just talk, talk, talk at these conferences, but it never turns into actual action that we could follow up with; it was an amazing conference.

JB: What other suggestions would you have for adults as to what can we do better as humans to help improve mental health?

SC: If you have a student, advocate at your school board meetings because I've seen how much power parents have at this amazing conference. This year, we had a parent panel, and their stories were so influential. Saying those types of things at the school board meetings influences how schools use the money that's coming down to them. And so essentially, you can be an advocate for your students' mental health and influence how that money is used to redirect it toward student mental health. Because every school needs to invest more in mental health. There's no escaping that need. And right now, there's a lot of money coming to schools but there's not a lot of usage of this funding or an understanding of how schools use funding; it's not clear whether there is follow through to see results.

JB: It feels like it needs to be consistent because it's not consistent. One school told me they had mental health week. One week in the whole year, and I thought, "That's nothing."

SC: Right. That's what it ends up being usually is a bunch of mental health clubs on campus, which we're very privileged to have, and just posters around the campus. At a certain point, just awareness is not enough. It needs to be followed up with that direct access to care on campus, which is why peer to peer is such an influential model.

JB: Definitely. I feel all the things that you've done during the pandemic have helped you in a lot of ways stay mentally strong.

SC: Taking action toward mental health makes sure that high school students who come after me will have something to rely on in terms of getting care on campus.

JB: And when you go off to college, you've got this toolkit of self-care and resilience and knowledge. Whereas some people going off to college don't always feel so strong.

SC: Yeah, and I'm hoping that our generation has that emphasis throughout their entire lives. So, self-care and mental health, we all go to college this year feeling more confident in our abilities and confident that we'll be able to adapt to this change.

Meet Kara Worrells

Manager, Artist, Researcher, Award-winning Poet

"Depression and anxiety became just as contagious as SARS-CoV-2 at the end of 2020.

For the first time in our global history, humanity could not deny that mental illness is everywhere. Everyone had life and death at the forefront of their thinking.

Everyone experienced meta panic and distress. We became active witnesses to chaotic suffering, forced to spectate the uncertainty of illness, even if we didn't want to be."

—Kara Worrells

Sometimes you meet someone by accident, but you quickly realize it wasn't an accident after all. I met Kara because we were both radio hosts at UC Irvine's station, KUCI 88.9 FM, and she reached out to ask about my show, my first book—*Get the Funk Out*—and my writing career. This chance encounter has turned into a friendship I truly treasure. Kara is extremely insightful, honest, resilient, incredibly wise, and a creative powerhouse. I have learned a lot from spending hours talking to her about life in a pandemic. Here's her take on why society was in a mental health crisis prior to March 2020, the outdated systems that don't work and never did, and how you have an important role in helping society become better humans.

Kara Worrells (KW): There's a lack of open, explicit conversation around emotion, around sensibility, and around what it means to be human in casual settings. Probably because we live in a society that regards certain topics as impolite to discuss in public and in private. Those topics include politics, religion, and any personal beliefs that could be considered disagreeable and inflammatory. This does not include willfully ignorant beliefs or hate speech, which I think is important to explicitly state because people can manipulate categorical associations to enable their insecurities and delusions. For example, the buzz-term "opinionated" is thrown around a lot to shame people into censoring their critical thinking about life and to discourage the thinking that reveals how complicated our simple lives actually are. We live in a world that reinforces a "don't ask, don't tell" culture, hypocritically, to shield sensibilities and prevent discomfort because socializing is meant to be casual, likable, enjoyable. Everyone is supposed to get along, even if it's only on the surface. It's not "that serious" even if it actually is, and vice versa, depending on the context.

I think we've been in a mental health crisis for centuries—since self-aware consciousness became a part of human existence, I'd argue. We've only recently acquired the language, beginning with twentieth-century psychology, to shed light on the different forms mental illness has taken for a long time. This realization in the twenty-first century comes from the vicious constant of mortality being in our faces. We can't look away. We can't deny the severity of individual suffering as it relates to the whole. We have been forced to continuously watch devastation, pain, and loss unfold on a global scale. Day in and day out, we've shared an intense horror over the threats of death and violence that have tortured every single one of our psyches. That trauma has taken root in every sphere of our lives. We are collectively defined by life after mass death. We are survivors of disaster.

It makes sense, then, that we'd call it a mental health pandemic. I think that title is a more accurate understanding of how an exponential pattern of mental health crises have evolved into a widespread, nondiscriminatory experience of struggle. Before COVID-19, it was more socially tolerable to be complacent, apathetic, and self-serving. An absence of accountability made corruption a home. We lived, and continue to live, in a world that rewards exploitation, manipulation, and subjugation. We live in a world that promotes the paranoia of "do it to them before they do it to you." Corruption is the norm. So, it makes sense why it was, and still is, challenging for people to truly trust and reel back their suspicions of one another in order to get healthy support.

Historically, the abuse of trust has caused a haunted need for healing. Planting the seeds of silence across generations has only furthered illness to take root, plague us, and sabotage our well-being. Talking about what causes us to experience sentiment is seen as a liability in a competitive world that is notorious, from its history, for building empires atop the destruction of neighboring communities by taking advantage of them from within. Supremacy is an unhealthy force that brings together foes instead of friends. So, it is considered safer to ignore feelings and deny vulnerabilities if questions of harm and power are in play.

I think that the coronavirus pandemic has given us an opportunity to be completely honest with our vulnerabilities and attachments, to be socially engaged with what unravels us and affects our senses, and to find protection in communities that value the fortitude of peaceful coexistence. The pandemic has reminded us of empathy and its strength. Empathy is the most powerful ability that humans have. To connect your thoughts with what your body experiences provides a reality check and a good reminder of what life is all about; it's like the concept of *The Body Keeps the Score* by Bessel van der Kolk. When we don't listen to how we feel, we neglect the logic of survival. We neglect this fundamental element of living that is directly communicating to us when we feel endangered versus when we feel safe. This is all rooted in trauma, abuse, and bullying. The toxic cycles of exploitative behavior keep us locked in emotional distress and mental harm. We have to get back to the root and review the fundamentals of why people do what they do, starting with the orchestrated stories that people tell themselves and one another.

Janeane Bernstein (JB): We started this conversation talking about a mental health crisis, mental health pandemic. Have you been struggling the entire time and before the pandemic?

KW: Yes, I've been struggling since I was about five years old, starting with depression. I saw a therapist temporarily when I was ten years old, and then I started therapy again in university. I should have had therapy day in and day out after I started struggling in elementary school, but I hope that the work I'm currently doing for my mental health will help me to find peace with accountability and the revelation of time.

Since I was a kid, mortality and suffering were constantly in my face, and they shaped who I am at my core. My empathy and care are all I am. I can see, in enduring this painful journey so far, that the only way through is to help other people as I help myself. Since I was a kid, I've wanted to pursue higher education. I've always been motivated by the intention to help other people in some way. As someone who pursues endless learning, self-reflection, and betterment, my family taught me that being of service would only be possible through education. I don't care about being the best; I care about being better than I was yesterday.

JB: We need to do better and be better as humans. And not everybody feels the same way you do. You are compassionate, empathetic, and people always don't walk through life like that. A lot of it has been "me, me, me." We are buried in our phones. People have a lot of apathy at times, and they don't act thoughtfully.

KW: It's exactly what the culture of the West is, specifically in the United States. This individualistic culture where, in order to be financially prosperous, to show off to other people, and to compensate for feeling inferior as a human being in society, you have to be selfish and project, project, project. You have to prioritize your desires, even if it's at the expense of other people's happiness, safety, stability, and truth. Ours is a culture of escapism that is perpetuated by capitalism, patriarchal abuse, and supremacist enforcement. We're not taking care of what we have and focusing on what's actually healthy and beneficial to us. There are false narratives about what's considered good because of what malicious people desire and enable as convenient, for example, social media and the spread of misinformation. It's like the game of "telephone," also known as "the grapevine." "I heard it from

TikTok" is commonly said nowadays. Numerous children in the United States died in 2018 from consuming poison just because it was popular. The hive mind and what it determines as desirable enable miseducation. Many people will believe what is not true and accept the temptation of trends without question if they are desperate to be involved.

Many will sacrifice independent thought, originality, and conviction because of fear—fear of being ostracized, of being seen as weird or different, of being bullied and physically threatened, or of being put down in a way where other people won't stand up for them because they themselves are afraid or apathetic. We have a deep-seated Stockholm syndrome that global society fears admitting to, but that's the first step in healing and recovery. We need to cut the bullshit and realize the truth. We need to talk about real, legislative solutions.

JB: When I heard how George Floyd died, with people standing around watching, it horrified me because I spent many years living in New York City where if something happened to someone, you ran over and helped. I didn't learn about the bystander effect there. I probably would have been arrested because I would have been yelling my ass off, and they would have charged me with obstructing justice.

KW: Exactly. How is it obstructing justice when you are killing people, these people who are peaceful and cooperative, in front of all of us? Trying to help prevent tyranny is not obstruction of justice; it's resisting the corruption of injustice. The enforcers of corrupt institutions manipulate rhetoric to create the illusion of legal legitimacy. They see themselves as above the law, capable of getting away with whatever they want, because they wear a badge, carry a gun, and cannot be physically touched without penalty of law.

History can have a cruel sense of humor. The police department is an institution that is rooted in White supremacy. Law enforcement was founded in the United States with the intention to protect slave owners in the South. Look up the article, "A Brief History of Slavery and the Origins of American Policing," written by Victor E. Kappeler. The United States has to own up to its history; that's where we have to start. We have to start with language and the words we choose to explain things. We have to start with reliable narrations of how we arrived in today's day and time because, with historical revision, we have to openly and correctly talk about these life events that we've inherited—in school, at home, with family, friends, people we agree with, and people we don't agree with. We have to be open, and we have to accept the responsibility of knowing the truth of what's been happening in our history. If we are tolerant of hate-motivated crimes and hate speech targeting marginalized communities, then we are tolerant of tyranny. We must be intolerant of superiority complexes. That's a collective duty. That's an individual duty.

I shared with Kara my strong feelings about mental health being embedded and prioritized into school curriculum, including strategies to promote conversations around mental health, wellness, and awareness.

JB: I feel that if we overhaul the curriculum in schools and build in mental health programs, workshops on an ongoing basis, it's going to alleviate the stress on teachers and counselors. It may create peer-to-peer moments for students to connect with one another and problem solve on issues. If it's escalated, obviously go to a counselor.

KW: Yeah, absolutely. This is standard conflict resolution. Mental health education is what we need to emphasize and prioritize because our psyches control everything in our lives. Our brains are the most powerful resource that we have available to us. Our government could do it today. No more wasting time and making excuses about the social politics of amending a curriculum. If our government wanted to, they could implement a straightforward mental health program for schools, today. They could do this as quickly as all of the legislative decisions they made in 2020 to address the coronavirus pandemic. We saw how fast they worked when death was right at their doorsteps; what is the difference in 2022 now that we have vaccinations to prevent potential death? The answer is in the question, so that's frustrating. Mindfulness and healthy coping skills aren't controversial, or at least they logically shouldn't be, so it shouldn't take them too long to offer our people the bare minimum, right? We have to think about the current events that are happening while we're alive and can do something about them. The people who choose to look away may feel like, no matter what they do, nothing will change. That they can't really do anything. So instead, to survive the circumstances, we assimilate. We adapt at the expense of our peace and say that "no news is good news" in order to relax, but futility buries justice.

The voice of the people is so often overlooked by those who have the power and money to make real-time, physical change that would improve our living conditions. It's understandable that it feels pointless and defeating to stand up for what we deserve, only to be tabled by government officials who believe they are rulers instead of service workers. The gatekeeping of comfortable, stable, and safe living is a frustrating dilemma that we are still resisting. It doesn't help the cause to improve our collective living when we don't organize our communities. Aren't we the people? We have to stand in our power and work together.

JB: So where do you think we go from here? The pandemic is making us wake up now. How do you think we can be better? Where do you think change needs to happen?

KW: We have to actively stay away from selfish lifestyles. We actively have to think about our choices; reflect on how we think and what we think about, especially since we're not always fully in control of our thoughts when they're affected by the environment and the abuse of language. So, in summary, we have to stay awake. We have to pay attention. We have to actively listen. We cannot succumb to mental laziness and excuses. We cannot allow ourselves to succumb to comfortable narratives, habits, or ways of living that serve gluttony and vanity. Boundaries with toxic behaviors and an intolerance of manipulation are crucial.

So, we start with ourselves and our thinking. Our inner voice—how we talk to ourselves and process experiences—can get stronger by reading, analyzing, and being critical of easy paths to what appears to be truth. Allowing other people's voices—their projections, their lack of insight and knowledge—to determine how you talk to yourself about life, affects everything. Knowing how to integrate and separate ourselves from one another is crucial. We all have to assume that responsibility and hold ourselves accountable so that as a collective, we can all heal. Healing means doing the groundwork of facing painful truths. We have to help ourselves so that we can help one another.

JB: How would you describe Gen Z? I'm asking because I admire your generation in that you're more open. You're more liberal. You're not afraid to say you need a mental health day, whereas someone my age…years ago, I probably would have never told you I'm going to therapy.

KW: I consider myself to be an in-betweener in life, in general, because of the complex identities that I assume. I identify as in between Gen Z and millennials since I was born in 1998.

I would say Gen Z is the most powerful generation that we have right now because they are the ones who are inheriting everything in our world. They are inheriting the earth. They are inheriting our social, legal, and economic institutions. They are inheriting narratives about life that are perpetuated in every social sphere. They're inheriting the education from our people in power—the knowledge that is made available to them with state-approved and federal-approved curriculums. They are inheriting everything. That makes Gen Z the most vulnerable.

They are the most vulnerable because they have yet to become fully independent. The youngest of the generation was born in 2012. It's 2022. Older adults still have a louder say in the lives that Gen Z gets to live. Knowing about the rise in physical, sexual, and psychological abuse against children and adolescents during the stay-in-place regulations set forth with the pandemic is especially horrifying. It's not enough to complain about it.

JB: Give me an example. You're even talking about Black Lives Matter.

KW: Yes, of course. A resurgence of Black Lives Matter protests began in April and May of 2020. It was at the forefront of dinner table conversations for some time, and then it got pushed once more to the back of people's minds. Life moved on from the public outcries, and people became numb to the violence once more. "That's life" is a phrase that's commonly said. People accept that abuse is a part of life because they do not believe it can be ended. Abuse doesn't follow any rules; it does what it wants. Innocent people end up getting hurt and living in the aftermath of violence because corrupt people will do anything to get their way. White supremacists, insecure with their bodies and identities, will do what they can to get rid of the people who remind them of their insecurities. They think that "out of sight" means "out of mind," but living in the residual world of the COVID-19 pandemic has proven otherwise.

Our government has yet to denounce the KKK. It's absurd that the United States would go to war with its own civilians who call for justice but will not condemn the White fragility that actively acts against Black lives. It's important to recognize that there are people who are doing the work. There are many people, like in the ACLU, who are making an active effort to protect our people. Every time I receive an email from the ACLU, I'm reminded of the good that is still going strong. There are people who are doing the work, but there are plenty of people who are not doing the work. People are comfortable in their bubbles. All of us need to act like a team. We have to do this with the mentality that we are all in this together, although there are plenty of people who want to sabotage this effort because of whatever self-serving agendas they have. That is what we have to be on the lookout for. We have to be on the lookout for people who sabotage. We have to keep an eye out for those who are not team members but who have decided to disguise themselves as such. We have to call it out. We have to be intolerant of that deception.

I can be patient and still uphold my moral and ethical beliefs; I'm not going to stand for certain behaviors to be permissible in the environments I enter, whether they're environments I have to enter or because I want to. I have to stay awake, and I have to be conscientious of actions as they have consequences. Whatever we do today is going to affect tomorrow. Whatever is present will stretch into the future. We have to constantly remind ourselves of cause and effect. Gen Z is the most vulnerable to our present actions. We have to be protectors. We cannot tolerate enablers.

Meet Rocket Garcia

Artivist

"That's where I'm at right now—just realizing that maybe I don't need to be fixed. Maybe the reason that I struggle with my feelings so much is because I'm still judging myself for having them."

—Rocket Garcia

I met Rocket when I attended a Los Angeles Youth Commission webinar in 2022. I was very moved by her personal journey and willingness to share her struggles and life lessons. Rocket is another creative dynamo who has a strong theater background, a passion to help marginalized communities, and endless creativity that shines in anything she puts her mind to, especially her cool TikTok videos!

Rocket Garcia (RG): When I was in K–12, nobody talked about mental health at all. I'm in college now, and it's definitely a little bit better, but I feel like most people just kind of dismiss young people's problems like, "You're not an adult yet, you don't really have actual issues." I feel like that can be really hard, and I'm still seeing that happen with young people. Today, it's like, "How hard can your problems actually be?" And just seeing people under eighteen, seeing them still struggling in ways that I definitely struggled at their age and still seeing it being written off as like, kind of cute or funny or not that serious. When in reality, I'm still dealing with the repercussions of not having my mental health taken seriously when I was a minor, under my parent's care. Because of that, I feel, and I'm twenty-three now and part of Gen Z, I'm moving forward in life.

Here's what Rocket shared about her mental health struggles prior to March 2020.

RG: I've been struggling with my mental health since I could process complex thoughts, or even basic thoughts. Some of my earliest memories are of me wriggling around and sobbing on the bathroom floor at the age of four or five. I felt like I was being pulled from the inside out. I would just sob and sob and try to hold my body together as a young child, which I later realized was anxiety. I was experiencing very intense anxiety from a very young age, and none of the adults in my life were really able to recognize that. I remember hearing, "She's just creative. She's just sensitive." But as I got older, my mental health struggles definitely continued to manifest more, and I would say become more debilitating in my life.

I would be bullied and known as the girl who cried for no reason by my peers in elementary school. I wouldn't eat, and

I learned to self-soothe through escapism, through the arts and reading. I would read constantly. I would go for walks as an elementary school student. I would leave. I would leave class when I felt overwhelmed and go for a walk. And it's so funny because you're not supposed to do that. I know a lot of schools that are more hardcore than the elementary schools I went to; they have a lot of guards posted and stuff, but somehow, I took my own agency. I think from a young age, I understood that no one was going to help me except me. And as I continued getting older, I started to have what I identified as panic attacks, like in high school, and I realized that maybe there was a reason why I was so creative, and was always drawing and knitting and doing other things in class, but I didn't receive any official diagnoses for anything I was going through until I was an adult. I know my mom did her best, but the adults in my life really failed me in that way.

Rocket was officially diagnosed at nineteen. She shared the following story on a Los Angeles County Youth Commission mental health panel that I attended. She described having anxiety while a student at Michigan College and what happened when she sought help. I hope no one ever experiences what Rocket had to endure, and may her story leave a mark on the minds and initiatives of mental health and wellness professionals within schools and college campuses.

RG: I went to a mental health counselor on campus. And at that point, I was just crying. I wasn't hysterical. Like I was just crying, and I told her I needed help. The woman was an absolutely horrible counselor. I needed her to just de-escalate the situation. I would have been fine if she'd just been like, "Hey, you know, maybe go home for the rest of the day. Like maybe rest, right?" Or even just ask me what's wrong? Like talk me through it. But as soon as she saw that I was in a state of panic, that I was crying, her first response was, "Let's get the police involved." And I don't know why. I don't know why that's what she meant. But that was a very, very traumatic experience for me, and that's when I really realized I got taken out of my life.

I asked her not to call the police, and I tried to calm myself down. And I did calm myself down, but it was too late. And she called the sheriff, and it was a tiny room. All of a sudden, I asked her, "If you have to call the police, can it at least be a woman?" Because I've had trauma, you know, with men. And she was like, "Okay," but there weren't any women sheriffs, and before I knew it, the room was flooded with like four or five male police officers. And they were chiding me and bullying me and harassing me into trying to make me say that I wanted to hurt myself, so that they could legally take me away.

Janeane Bernstein (JB): Oh, come on!

RG: Yeah, they kept asking me over and over again, "Do you want to hurt yourself? Do want to hurt yourself? Don't kill yourself." And I was like, "Bro, bro, bro, like, no. No." And ultimately, they got me to confess that I had self-harmed in high school. Because of their incessant bullying, because legally in order to 5150 somebody, legally, it doesn't matter if they were suicidal yesterday. Doesn't matter if they were suicidal three days ago and has to be in that moment. You have to have proof that they wanted to harm themselves or someone else in that moment.

JB: But there wasn't any proof. Is that what a 5150 is?

RG: Yes. A 5150 is when the police are legally able to remove you from your life and put you into a mental institution against your will. And that's what happened to me. I had a panic attack on campus at school. I went to look for help. Wound up having the police called on me, and they took me away. And I was forcibly put into a mental health institution, which was absolutely terrifying. You know, I did the whole "squat and cough thing." [They] took all my clothes, my phone, [and I] couldn't call anybody except through their phone and couldn't have visitors except for one hour in the evening and on a specific day. Mom couldn't even come see me when it happened. I was just all by myself.

JB: How long were you there?

RG: Fortunately, I was only there for like a day and a half. Well, the first thing that happened was the police actually took me to a regular hospital. And they were like "a psychiatrist is going to come check you out. And if they think that you're okay, you're free to go home." But there's only at least at that time, which was just a few years ago, there were only three psychiatrists for the entire LA County who hop around from hospital to hospital, checking in on folks who been detained for mental health reasons. Three. And of course, none of the three were able to see me, so I got transferred to the mental health institution in the middle of the night. They strapped me down in the ambulance; it was absolutely terrifying. I think I was like freshly nineteen. I was just out of high school; it was crazy. And there was no one to advocate for me because I moved out here away from my family. As a young person, I didn't feel comfortable and didn't know how to advocate for myself. Yeah, I didn't know my rights. I wasn't allowed to feel like I had any rights, you know? And I was just made to feel like I was crazy, and I was being transported around and it was just insane. Once I got there, I had to take all my clothes off. I had to do the squat and cough and they took all my stuff. And I just looked around me and I was like, "This is horrible."

The way that mental health institutions are depicted in *One Flew Over the Cuckoo's Nest* is still applicable. Nothing's really changed. They were so convinced everyone in there was on medication that the nurse came up to me in the morning and she's like, "Have you taken your meds?" And I was like, "I'm not on any meds." She was like, "No, but have you taken them?" And I was like, "I don't have any meds." And she didn't believe me, and she had to go check. We weren't treated well. It was very, very weird. I read the entire pamphlet of what they're supposed to be able to provide for us. They were supposed to be able to provide us with envelopes and pencils and paper so that we could write letters, and I asked them for that. And they didn't have any of that. But yeah, so that was that was my big experience that showed me I cannot rely on the systems that are in place. It really made me feel like I have to hide that next time.

I asked Rocket what she would do differently if she could experience this situation all over again. I wondered if she would have gone to anyone for help?

RG: I wouldn't have gone to anyone. I would have suppressed it. It was absolutely terrifying. To this day, I have a lot of traumas around police for multiple reasons, but some people don't believe you, and a lot of people know. It doesn't matter what you do. People in power can choose—like police officers can just choose to take you away. If I get pulled over, I make sure I'm extremely calm, because I know they'll use any excuse to put you somewhere if they don't want to deal with you.

JB: So, do you have any idea what brought on that anxiety attack that morning?

RG: Yeah, I was doing a lot. I was just overwhelmed. I was involved in three musical productions at the time. I was doing school. I had a lot to take care of, and what triggered that particular attack was that I had a rehearsal to go to, and I hadn't practiced what I said I would because I didn't have time. I just took that really hard, and that tends to be one of my main triggers—when I feel like I'm not doing well enough.

JB: Have you learned anything about this experience in taking better care of yourself?

RG: Yeah, 100 percent. I think it's a constant struggle for me because as someone who does have ADHD and who has grown up with feeling like I'm already a couple steps behind, I tend to push myself really hard. I tend to be somebody who is chronically overbooked. But part of what's been amazing about my journey, and I think what's really helped me with this, is the environment that I'm in now. I no longer do theater. I'm more involved. It's funny. I'm more involved in activist spaces now, and my job, which is very focused on ancestral teachings, has helped me really feel part of a community with others and learn more, and to feel more free to explore my own indigenous heritage. It's just really helped me to move away from these colonial mindsets of constant productivity, that my self-worth is based on what I do, and that's something that I have slowly been working through, and that's what's allowed me to do some of my own healing and have fewer panic attacks; it's just giving myself more slack, really.

JB: That's great. And it sounds like you are connecting with something meaningful and purpose driven as opposed to a paycheck and a title and a "GO GO GO!" attitude. Do you feel that what you do has provided a little bit of healing, as far as a sense of connection, a sense of purpose?

RG: Yes! (Laughter) My whole life, I was so convinced that there's something really wrong with me. And I'd say that I felt that way even up to a few days ago.

JB: Really?

RG: Yes! (Laughter) I only very recently started this new art of radical self-acceptance because of a conversation I had with my mentor, and I was expressing to her. I was in one of my spaces where I'm sobbing uncontrollably because that's something I still struggle with. It still affects my day-to-day life. I was sobbing uncontrollably. I was like, I don't know what to do. I don't know what to do.

JB: With your life or with this crying?

RG: I don't know what to do with myself because I've been going through a breakup. My mom has been wanting to be there for me. But the way that my parents are there for me is they're like, "This isn't normal. Like, what you're going through isn't normal. The way you're living isn't normal. And we need to figure out what's wrong to fix you." My room was really messy. I'm not in classes this semester. And I have really intense meltdowns, and she was saying we need to get you like checked out neurologically; this has been ignored for too long. And I've been going through this process my whole life, you know. I was expressing this to my mentor, and I was like, I don't know what to do. Because when I'm struggling and when I turn to the people that I feel like I can trust, they always make me feel worse.

JB: Yes, like you have to be "fixed." They said, "We have to fix you."

RG: Yeah. And where I'm at right now is just realizing that maybe I don't need to be fixed. Maybe the reason that I struggle with my feelings so much is because I'm still judging myself for having them.

JB: Oh, yes. That's a tremendous insight. Because there is that negative self-talk on a loop. People do it of all ages. I can see where you would think that. I know you're a writer, but do you have any kind of physical outlets, or are you musical? What do you love to do?

RG: I love to do everything. And that's what's so sad about mental health. I feel like as a child, I was able more freely to turn to the arts when I needed to self-soothe. I feel like I have gotten to a point where sometimes I'm so, so sad. And I'm so tired and so drained that I really don't feel like I can do anything. But what's fortunate lately is that I'm not in that headspace. And what I like to do is I love making TikToks! (Laughter)

JB: Yes, I have seen some of them! They are really good!

RG: (Laughter) You have seen my TikToks? Okay, well, I make TikToks. And I love writing songs. I used to write musicals a lot and actually have had most of my musicals produced. Since I'm not really doing theater anymore, I've realized that the songs that I write don't have to be in a musical. They can be standalone songs. I do like writing songs. I draw. I go for walks every day. My psychiatrist prescribed mental health walks. Some of the TikToks I make are like, taking people along with me on my mental health walks because it always inspires me to see other people doing what I want to do. I want to help others who may be struggling to find that inspiration. And then I knit. I cook. I crochet. I sew. I love video games. Very challenging video games are actually surprisingly very stress relieving for me. It's good. I like everything. I'll try anything really.

JB: Well, I could tell when I asked the question because your whole face lit up talking about this.

RG: It's my favorite thing to do. Doing stuff is my favorite part of life.

JB: If you were in charge of school policy or to make changes, you've got STEM and STEAM, but I don't really think mental health has been integrated into the curriculum the way it should be. But if you were going into schools, if you were going to make changes, what would you like to see done differently?

RG: Well, first of all, the entire policies around truancy would be completely different. I missed so much school growing up. I was a truant, and if it wasn't for my mom being on top of paperwork and stuff, I probably would have gone to juvie, and she probably would have gotten into trouble as well. I missed a lot of school. And it was always because I felt like I could not do it. And I think that I've actually thought about this before. I know a lot of kids really struggle with truancy because they're going through home issues and that affects their mental health and all kinds of stuff. The first thing I would do is I would make it less abrupt, especially for young people or for anyone with neurodivergent brains.

We really struggle with transitioning, especially someone who has ADHD. Transitioning from task to task is very challenging. I would make school start later because everyone I knew growing up was chronically exhausted. Kids have to wake up way too early, especially with their growing bodies and minds. We need more rest. So, school would start later. The first period would be maybe thirty minutes of transitioning, and this applies across the board. I'm talking K–12. The first period would be a transition, like "Let's have some time to reflect on how we are showing up to school today. And do we want to share that?" It's okay if you don't and if you do. So that like it's not so abrupt, like "Get in the car! Get in the car! Let's go!"

Like just having a little bit of time to transition. I think that would be very helpful, and then just funding for the arts is mandatory. So many schools don't get the funding they need. Those are the first programs that get cut. Every single child needs to have access to a creative outlet. And these programs are the most important thing. If I hadn't had access to the arts programs that I did growing up, I'm sure I'd be in a lot more trouble than I am now; that's just so important. So, I feel these are the main things. School would start later. Youth would have a chance to transition into their day, and mandatory funding for the arts. And then the last thing would be there would not be any police on campus. They would be replaced with community teams, which are actually called the Yes teams. That goes into Youth Justice Reimagined, which is a project I've been working on, but I would not have the police on campus.

Here are Rocket's ideas for preventative programming, mental health workshops, and activities geared towards student resilience.

RG: I would definitely advocate for actual licensed therapists on campus, and multiples of them. Like enough to handle not just two or three [students], which tends to be the case. Yeah, 100 percent. That's actually such a great question, because I remember feeling like many times that no one would help me unless it got to a point where they couldn't ignore it anymore. And I think what's really important to be part of that is making sure every child has their own plan in place, you know what I mean? Like, "What can I do if I'm having a hard day," because there may be a point where every day is a hard day and maybe they'll have that guidance from adults in their lives, from the community; they'll have a plan in place. So, they're not just floundering, when it happens.

JB: I know we're in a mental health pandemic. Suicide rates have gone up, anxiety, depression, et cetera. What do you think are the factors that have affected mental health? Can you think of things in your life or others' lives that have caused the spike in these issues?

RG: The main thing is the isolation and getting taken out of your life. I've seen, especially among people my age, that the isolation really affected us badly, and a lot of my friends are still struggling. I know that will probably be a trauma that we will carry with us for the rest of our lives. Every time [I listen to] the news, there's like a "We might have to go into quarantine again." I'm like, I'd actually rather die (laughter). I would rather die than have to not see anyone for months on end the way that we did, except for the folks that we live with.

JB: Because it's detrimental. It's detrimental to be socially isolated.

RG: It's extremely detrimental and it makes you feel like you're alone. And I think that a lot of us were going through very similar things. But we felt even more alone than usual. It's already so challenging to talk about what you're going through, and the fact that we weren't even around anyone to talk about or see how each other was doing. I think that there's many factors to this, but I would say the isolation is the main one. And then especially for our relatives who are in the LGBT community, we have to acknowledge that the suicide rates are much higher among trans youth of color. I speak to this with my acknowledgment that there are definitely folks who could speak to this better because I am not a trans person. [I can only say this] knowing my friends and knowing what they've gone through, [including] just being in an environment where you're getting dead-named, day after day, where you don't have that escape to school.

For those of you who don't know what *dead-named* is, I asked Rocket to explain:

RG: Being dead-named is when somebody uses a dead name—basically the name that a trans person was born with. For example, someone was assigned female at birth, and their name was Trudy. They later realized, "This is not my gender identity, and this is not me."

JB: And they want to be called Troy.

RG: And they changed their name to Troy.

JB: And people are still intentionally calling them Trudy to hurt them?

RG: It doesn't matter if it's intentional or not, it's still dead naming, because the effect is still the same. It can still cause gender dysphoria. And so, I think that's another major factor. There's a lot of young people who are trapped in these situations where their identities are not being respected, where they're not allowed to feel safe to live as they are. And, you're in this place where "It's okay, the pandemic will be over in a month, two months, three months, two years..." and it starts to feel like nothing's ever going to change. I completely understand why many young people are taking their lives because there were several times during the pandemic where I felt such intense despair. I mean, I was pretty safe, compared to other folks. I was pretty safe during the pandemic, in terms of my living situation. And there were a couple times where I just was like, this is never going to end.

And that's the thing. I feel like older people, for whatever reason, were better able to think in their heads, "Well, this isn't going to last forever, you know," but I saw a lot in my generation, that despair and that hopelessness, of not being convinced that this wouldn't end. I think that's part of it as well. So, it's the isolation factor, being unsafe, like in housing situations, being in situations where you're not safe to be yourself, where you don't feel free to be yourself, where your identity is constantly being rejected or even worse, ridiculed. And then also, we haven't been alive as long as y'all, and so just having less context of like being in the world. It's a lot easier to think, "Well, damn, it's been like this for a while. Maybe this is just how things are now, and I can't live like this."

JB: Would that be part of policy changes in schools? To educate people on the correct way to care about one another?

RG: I don't think that everything can be on schools; there's so much that schools already need to do differently in terms of education. I think that comes from community support, not just your family and your school, but also some type of activity or group that connects you with your community. Whatever community that might be.

Rocket shared her thoughts on what the pandemic has taught society about being better humans, and other lessons that can be learned:

RG: Here's the thing. I think people are going to be how they're going to be. Yes, you can educate and that can definitely make a huge difference, but at the end of the day, people are free to be assholes if they want to. So, I would say that if there is a lesson to be learned, it's that we need to deconstruct our systems and how they have been structured for White straight cis men, and just recreate, just reimagine the culture around what we expect of ourselves and each other and allow each other to be human. I think that's really the main lesson; it's not healthy or sustainable to act like a machine. We all have different needs, and there isn't a systematic way to take care of everybody's needs. We have to feel secure enough and whatever foundation to allow people to be flexible; that's something that I really feel is modeled well at my place of employment. I've been very grateful for that if I do have to call out of work sometimes because I can't pull it together. I'm so fortunate to have a job like that because I have had jobs that weren't like that. Not everyone is fortunate enough to have that, but we have to be less focused on what's the profit going to be like, what's the bottom line, and more focused on just allowing each other to function like we need to.

Rocket shared her views on the functions of society and the role it has in addressing the mental health pandemic.

RG: At the end of the day, the whole point of society is to keep everyone safe, right? The whole point of even having a society and a government is to make sure that people's basic needs are taken care of and [have] strength in numbers. A government was established to protect the people. The way that things are established, they're not to protect the people; they are to protect the money.

We will continue to be in a mental health pandemic unless we completely shift the way our society is run. And I think that can be said for every single issue that we see today. We will still always have a climate change issue if we don't completely overhaul the way our current system is run. We will always have a systemic racism issue if we don't completely overhaul. You see what I'm saying? And so, the way our society is functioning right now is—it is not. Everyone is struggling. Some people are just better at masking it than others. I mean, maybe there's one guy (laughter) who's in his yacht in Florida sipping on a mojito and he's happy, but none of us are well until all of us are well. So yeah, I would just say the main lessons we learned from this is we can't expect ourselves to go on this way. Because it's not right.

JB: And it's not working.

RG: And it's not working. I think that part of the problem is that we live in such an individualistic culture that compounds the isolation—so kind of moving away from individualism into collectivism. [We have to] let go of that myth that we can't be loved until we love ourselves. I just think that's so wrong. We do need to feel loved. How are you going to learn to love yourself if you've never experienced love from someone else? So just like letting go of that whole, hyper-independent, "I have to take care of this. This is my problem. I'm struggling with my mental health, and I need to be fixed and no one come near me." It perpetuates that isolation. Think of what people need. I think people need to know that. They're going to be accepted. They're not going to be shunned by society for having problems. I think struggles—that's just part of being human. We have struggles and, being able to know, "I do still have worth because I'm a human being," and continuing to build that trust with yourself and build that self-confidence and self-esteem by acknowledging I am contributing, whether that being through like creating art, creating something where there was nothing, or delivering the bagels that would have been thrown away. I think a big part of that also is being able to share what you're doing with others.

Meet Zach Faerber

Community Builder, Sales Enthusiast, Owner of Faerber Fitness

"Right alongside with mental health is cherishing your gifts, being more emotionally in tune and knowing you're not the only one. It's okay to be sad. It's okay to be depressed, anxious, whatever you're feeling is fine. Just make sure you're not doing it alone, and make sure that you have your circles."

—Zach Faerber

I have known Zach for years and was friends with his mother, Toni, who was from the same hometown as my grandmother. Toni passed away in 2015, just two days before my father died. Zach was born and raised in Orange County, California, and moved all over California after he lost his beloved mother to cancer. He now resides in San Diego. We have had numerous conversations over the years, and I am honored he agreed to share his story.

Janeane Bernstein (JB): I remember when we last spoke. You were in the operating room, assisting on different procedures.

Zach Faerber (ZF): Knee replacements. It's really interesting how when we were speaking it was such an integral part of my journey of grief, of mental health, getting back to me. I thought I had figured it out, but I was still deep in the negative coping mechanism. I was working in medical devices, and I transitioned to trauma because I was like, "I want to impact more people. I want to help." And it ended up making me lose my mind. I was working eighty to a hundred hours a week. I would get calls at midnight to two in the morning about cases and go to the hospital, and then that transitioned into COVID. The hospitals were impossible to get into. There was a ton of poor decisions being made by our doctors, on our end and on the staff. Nurses didn't want to come into work. Nobody knew how to protect themselves. I remember standing outside of an operating room because I wasn't allowed in because it was a COVID case. No one had indicated it was a COVID case so somebody could have just walked in. I was walking and talking to the nurse inside to tell them what implants to grab, what to set up for the doctor, and then one of the COVID Safety Specialists accidentally bumped the door open. All of a sudden, everybody's running and I'm standing there. Long story short, I got COVID twice. I was out of commission for about seven days. I lost nine pounds. I woke up one morning to three hundred phone calls. My anxiety was through the roof, and I was not making a crazy amount of money. I wasn't happy even if I was making a crazy amount of money. It's not worth it.

JB: I bet you didn't have much time to work out and take care of yourself.

ZF: I'd go through those very circular patterns, waking up at four in the morning, go to the gym for a week, prep meals, and then crash and burn and sleep through the alarm for twelve hours on my one day. I'd have to be in surgery. I wasn't sleeping much. I wasn't eating much; it takes getting to that point before you can rebound.

My parents were sick for so long, and that was my mentality. I'm going to work three jobs. I'm going to do bodybuilding. I'm going to play ice hockey. I'm going to work out. There's so much jampacked into your life that you don't have a moment to step back, take a breath, and go, "Well, what am I dealing with right now? What's going through me?" I have enough hours of therapy to be a therapist myself. It wasn't until recently that I found other kinds of modalities, and it's so funny because growing up in Orange County, my dad and my mom had a very conservative household. And now I'm here doing breathwork ceremonies and just getting out of my comfort zone and it's refreshing. I did my first hour of breathing, which is so counterintuitive to me because I do it all the time, but deep breathing [is different]. I haven't cried like that in so long. It was very beautiful to let yourself sit with something, then unravel it and understand what are those traumas that I'm holding on to, whether it's childhood or something that I've been telling myself for a while now. I just understand that they're there. That's kind of mind blowing.

I just feel so much more at ease and relaxed and at peace with things, and I think that you need to get to that place. And a lot of people say I don't have time, or I don't want to do breathwork, but it's like with anything—you need to make time.

JB: I want to rewind. Before we started, I asked if we could talk about this. Years ago, I remember I went to the service for your dad because he had cancer.

ZF: He had cancer four times. [He had] remission four times before; it wasn't even cancer that killed him. There was something called graft versus host disease; it's with blood cancers. He had non-Hodgkin's lymphoma. Once you run out of those treatment options, they actually recommend a stem cell transplant, which is somebody else's or your own.

October 31, 2006 was a hard day to forget. We're running around in our Halloween costumes, and he went through surgery because he had some pain in his spleen. They were going to take out his spleen, and they found cancer, so he went through his first round of chemo. He went into remission, and then he would just wake up with a tumor the size of a golf ball on the side of his face or on his chest; it was crazy. I remember him coming home after the third round of cancer being in remission—bald, no eyebrows, and he disappeared for like eight hours and we were all freaking out. He came home, and he had this huge tattoo of like a scroll with dogs and the date each day he went to remission, and I was like that's so silly. And unfortunately, he got it again. But it was just so interesting to see how he was coping. He passed from graft versus host switch, which is like, when you give stem cells, there's still a chance that your body rejects them and fights it. So, then your body pretty much kills itself because it rejects the new cells. He passed May 28, 2011, which is my aunt's birthday, unfortunately.

JB: What did getting a tattoo do for you—mentally or emotionally?

ZF: It's almost like associating pain with the situation. And then when it's done, it almost felt like this emotional release that helped me move through that and since then, I've gotten more. After my mom passed, I got a huge rose on my side for her, and it was the same feeling. I waited six months after I got it, and I just felt like this stage of grief moving through it.

My brother and my sister all have LUB, standing for "love you best." My mom used to say it to us. We all have that matching—"love you best."

JB: That's beautiful. I have such good memories of your mom. I remember her car with the big eyelashes.

ZF: That was her dream because we had a puppy. We got a puppy, and her dream was always to have a Mini Cooper and our puppy. I was just talking to someone about the community. I had a lot of mental health stuff going on and the community—you guys were what really propped me up and it really taught me that being alone is a choice. It's a hard choice to get yourself out of, right? It's not easy, but there are a billion people on this planet. If you reach out, there are people like yourself and people in this community that will have open arms. The beauty in the lesson for me was creating that community; it's so important to me in my life and my journey forwards. So, I don't know if I've ever gotten the chance to thank you for everything you do and have done absolutely goes for everybody—any big part of that Orange County Jewish community. Thank you.

JB: Well, I remember I wanted to do something, and somebody said, "We're starting a meal train." I signed up.

Other people signed up, and we would just show up with coolers of food.

ZF: You can't imagine how much it meant to have a warm meal when she was getting sick at the end; it was just such a ray of sunshine.

I asked Zach to take me back to after his dad passed away, and to share where he was mentally and emotionally. I told him to share whatever level of detail he was comfortable with. As expected, he went through a really difficult time. I remember attending his dad's funeral, and the community was rocked to the core. I wanted to see whether losing his dad and what happened after made him more resilient to address struggles he had the past few years.

ZF: Yeah, it's very interesting. I think it goes back to me and to that aloneness. You feel that isolation, that loneliness, and [I think] the pattern is there for a lot of people right now. When my dad was really sick, I was suicidal. I did make a couple of attempts, and on one of them, my mom found me and helped me. I basically dropped out of high school at the time, and she helped me get into a program that really helped.

At first, they were trying to push things and trying to get me on the right medication for my hormones or whatever and eventually connected me with one of the therapists that really helped me work on my coping mechanisms, and that kind of led me to where I am now. But yes, the similarities from that feeling, that depth of isolation and aloneness, could very well be felt during COVID. I'd come home working that many hours just mentally and physically exhausted, and just break down. I had a hard time crying for the longest period after my parents passed away. Recently, I've been able to kind of release in that way, but it was just a lot of anger, a lot of anxiety, a lot of throwing myself into more work, throwing myself into more unhealthy habits. You know, I did go down the drug route for a little while, but nothing too crazy, but sure, I was still trying to numb with those substances.

If somebody had said to me, "Go easy on yourself," I think people just need to hear that right now. You're going through so much. It's all valid. Whatever you're feeling is valid. That feeling of being resilient and dealing with so much at such a young age, all of a sudden, like numbs the smaller things. So, I'll get rear ended and I'm like, whatever. It's not a big deal. Just give yourself a break. Take a minute. Take a breath and look at all you're doing. It may not feel like a lot, especially adding in work from home. All of a sudden, your workspace becomes your life space. It all starts to bleed together. Yes, people tend to forget that we are not our work.

Zach shared the impact of the pandemic on him personally and on society. He is optimistic and hopeful that there are lessons to be learned that can be a catalyst for change.

ZF: This (the pandemic) is something that nobody has ever in the history of humanity experienced before, this kind of depth of new lifestyle so quickly. On the other hand, we have the chance to really stop and look at these statistics and look at these articles and say, "What can we do right now?" and just start chipping away. I'm very hopeful that we're getting to that point where people are starting to wake up and realize this may be how life continues. We will always have some sort of a byproduct of COVID. Let's figure out how to live healthy and sustainably while living with it. Conversations are starting to trend toward mental health and understanding how you can be the best version of yourself and then add work on top of prioritizing yourself. I think those conversations are going to start happening more and more because we've been about consumption and productivity for so long.

Zach shared advice for people who are struggling with their mental health. He knows from experience how difficult it is to take the first step and acknowledge you need help, but once you do, you will begin to have a change in perspective. He also finds that helping others is a great way to help yourself.

ZF: Make that choice to get out of your comfort zone just a bit—put your hand up so that somebody can at least see you and be there for you. I think my biggest issue in the moment was not that anybody cared. It's just so not true. There are people who care, and I make it as easy as possible for people to try to communicate with me—for people to book time on my calendar to communicate. Just having a thirty-minute conversation can really change your perspective on things. Just try to have a conversation with someone trying to go out of your way. Once you do get into the position where you're going to volunteer and do something for somebody else, you experience a perspective shift and give in; it changes in the giving in, and it's priceless. It's so easy to do and so rewarding.

JB: You went from working in an emergency room, not getting asleep, and working your butt off to now having a more peaceful, more fulfilling, well-rounded life.

ZF: I think once you start working on yourself, it's a never-ending journey. I feel way more aligned with what fills me up. Just look at your priorities. Look at where you're spending your time and if they're aligned. What do you want to do every day? What makes you feel good? Because now, more than ever, there's more ways to do more, make and sustain and live off of nonprofits, off of whatever you want to do.

Whatever you want to be and bring into this world, there's somebody who's done it. There's somebody who can show you how to do it, and there's a way to make it happen. So, if you feel out of alignment, it's your body telling you it's time to find your purpose. And it shifts all throughout.

One thing I'd love to bring up is I felt so self-conscious and self-aware. I hated myself for a long time for being a sensitive man, for being someone who has emotions. Yeah, especially when I was younger. You're supposed to be tough, especially going through what I did. You know, [as a] man of the house, [you're supposed to] "GO DO DO DO!" And I always kind of stored that away. But I've always been sensitive. I've always been emotionally more attuned with myself, and that's something that I looked down on for so long. And I know a ton of other men that I've met that are not willing to open up; they're not willing to go there because it looks like a weakness, but there are spaces for that, and there is so much opportunity to let that flourish and let that be you. I think it goes right along with mental health because for so long, I was living out of alignment, thinking I have to be this macho bodybuilder. I can't be sensitive or anxious or whatever. I tend to be the life of the party when I go to parties. I love to entertain and have friends, but I have crippling social anxiety, and people would have never guessed that.

The next chapter will feature voices from teachers and educators, their personal and professional struggles, and insights into how schools and policymakers should prioritize mental health initiatives. I am thankful to those who were so candid and willing to share their experiences and opinions in a time of personal and professional upheaval.

CHAPTER 5

The Pandemic Life of Teachers and Educators

"People are leaving in high rates. It's a really hard time to be a teacher and to be a counselor, and these are adults who have put themselves on the frontlines, in terms of exposure, many times to the virus; and also, are trying to support students without having the resources that they need."
—*Dr. Jennifer Greif Green, associate professor in special education, Boston University Wheelock College of Education & Human Development*

Consider for a moment what it has felt like to be a teacher in the United States in a pandemic. For teachers and educators reading this, I tried to fathom the mental, physical, and emotional toll of the pandemic on your lives, having to shift to online learning, adhere to safety protocols, staff shortages, political debates over what can and cannot be discussed in the classroom, handling the faceless black screens of students, and struggling to keep students engaged. Then faced with more news of school shootings, feeling underappreciated and undercompensated, and seeing students crumble emotionally and academically. And if your world wasn't stressful enough, some of you experienced the chaos of TikTok challenges, like the "Slap

Your Teacher Challenge," which TikTok spoke up about. No one prepared you for life as a teacher during a pandemic, and my heart goes out to you.

On the flip side, you might have noticed more students reaching out to you because they were struggling with their mental health. Students did not always feel comfortable connecting with their parents, so they turned to teachers and other adult figures for help. Adding to your role as a teacher or educator, you suddenly became a counselor, a mentor, and a life coach. Your lives also included juggling your own roles and responsibilities as a parent, while dedicating hours to preparing online instruction that might not have been received because all you were seeing were a plethora of black screens where student faces should have been. You had no idea if they were comprehending your material and how they were coping mentally and emotionally. The amount of pivoting, shifting, and increase in your workload and stressors was not always recognized and addressed; it's no wonder there was an enormous exodus of teachers from the field. Your mental health was challenged like never before.

On August 12, 2022, Yahoo News featured Rebecca Pringle, the president of the National Education Association (NEA), the largest teachers' union in the country. She shared details of the teacher shortage crisis. Pringle said it wasn't new, but the pandemic exacerbated the problem. When I read the alarming number of teacher and school staff vacancies, I took a double take and had to read it again—three hundred thousand. Let that number sink in for a moment.

With students going back in person, there was concern that they would not receive the attention they needed. Pringle pointed out that there are even more Black and Latina teachers planning to leave. When asked how to address this problem, she said: "One of the things that I've learned from educators—I traveled all over the country, from Kentucky to California to Maine to Wisconsin to Illinois—and they all said the same thing. This is what they need to come into the profession and stay in the profession. They need professional respect." Pringle said this means, "Professional authority to make teaching and learning decisions for their students. Professional rights to have the conditions and resources to do the jobs they love. And professional pay that reflects the importance of the work they do."

The life of a teacher also included tremendous anxiety and stress over school shootings. Becoming a teacher should not feel as if you are going off to a war zone where schools must now install metal detectors like airports, have active shooter drills (imagine what this feels like for children and how they process that experience), encourage teachers to carry guns, and where students and teachers live in fear and trauma instead of enjoying school as a place of learning, safety, meaningful relationships, creativity, and play.

The pandemic shined a light on just how important our mental health is. It emphasized that mental health should be talked about and destigmatized. Proper training and education must be provided so people know who to reach out to, how to properly care for those struggling, how to prioritize their own mental health, and what staff and resources must be available to address the needs of those suffering. Teachers already had a full plate to begin with, but then the pandemic caused incredible stress and added mental health duress to the mix.

Consider the following:

- What is the ripple effect of a teacher shortage?
- Who is looking out for the mental health of teachers?
- Do teachers have mental health resources and access to support *their* mental and emotional health, while managing the mental health of students?
- Are teachers appreciated, respected, and supported by their school administrators, parents, and students?

- Are teachers trained and educated in how to help students who are struggling with their mental health? Do they know the warning signs and appropriate steps to take?
- When college students are studying to become a teacher, does the teacher preparation curriculum support student mental health with peer-to-peer experiences, clubs, programs, and workshops to prioritize the mental health of students that will soon be facing a critical and challenging career choice? Do they feel they have a foundation to support their mental health as teachers in training and knowledge and skills that they can use in the future?
- Do these students feel they have a community and support system within their schools?

The next section includes conversations with several insightful teachers and educators who took the time to share their views on the global mental health pandemic, their thoughts on becoming better humans, and what challenges they have faced the past few years. You can listen to the full versions of these conversations on my podcast: www.otbseries.com.

I am honored to have met:

- *Jessica Alejandro*—Graduate student and teacher, New York City
- *Dr. Jennifer Greif Green*—Associate Professor in Special Education, Boston University Wheelock College of Education & Human Development
- *Octavio Hernandez*—Middle school teacher and board member, Polk Education Association, Florida
- *Ross Gothelf*—Eleventh grade Civics & Economics teacher, Denver, Colorado
- *Oleksandr Elkin*—A Ukrainian public figure and the founder of the responsible teaching movement, EdCamp Ukraine

- *Dr. Michael Yassa*—Professor of Neurobiology and Behavior, Neurology and Psychiatry at University of California Irvine, Director of the Center for the Neurobiology of Learning and Memory

Meet Jessica Alejandro

Graduate student and teacher, New York City

"I always say our students carry more in their backpacks than their books and their pencils.

"They carry these mental health issues that we go through as adults. They carry with them neglect and abuse. They carry things that we may know of and a lot we may not know of. There were times that I needed someone through my depression and grief, and I want to be there for my students."

—Jessica Alejandro

Jessica is a graduate student at Queens College, City University of New York (CUNY), studying Elementary Special Education. She is a substitute teacher at a New York City Department of Education Elementary School and is the New York City Team Lead for the national COVID memorial organization, Yellow Heart Memorial. She is a mental health advocate and was one of Mental Health America's 2022 conference speakers. Her workshop, "Coping with COVID: Using Grief to Create Change," was virtually viewed by over four hundred people as she spoke about the loss of her grandfather to COVID in March 2021 and how she and her sister were helping those within the COVID community in his memory.

Jessica recently spoke at a Mental Health America conference in DC. When I heard about her and her willingness to share her story of loss and resilience, I reached out to connect. We have spent hours chatting about everything from mental health to sharing laughs and thoughts on life. I can't wait to meet her in person one of these days.

Jessica Alejandro (JA): I feel like not only has the pandemic definitely hindered our ability to be a part of different spaces where we can share things, but I feel like a lot of us mentally during the pandemic had to face the things that we were avoiding in our lives. Our mental health, of course, has deteriorated so much that it was very hard for us to share the things that we've gone through with people who may not understand, may not want to understand, may be in a mindset that, you know, "Oh, I've heard this before," or that "You're not depressed. You're sad. Everybody's going through it. You're just sad."

I graduated with my BA during the pandemic. My graduation ceremony was a pre-recorded YouTube video. So, of course at that time, it was so horrible for me.

Janeane Bernstein (JB): Depressing! I worked this hard for this?!

JA: Fast forward to today where they had their in-person ceremonies and everything and our class 2020 and 2021 weren't even acknowledged. So, it was like, "You're fine. You graduated."

JB: No, no. That's horrible.

JA: Yes, and I am glad other colleges didn't do that. I know of a few who were allowing people for the past few years to walk or even just acknowledge them in some way, shape, or form, but it was a lot for us and then people were getting sick. Family members [were] getting sick, myself losing my grandpa last year. Trying to do school at the same time when not really having friends. Or if I did have people, I didn't want to feel like a burden and still don't want to feel like a burden when I'm having my depressive moments. Because I have heard, "You're not depressed, you're just sad," or "You just need to go out and get some air or you have to do this…" especially with depression. I have found that everybody seems to have a one quick fix. Slap a Band-Aid on it. "Alright, you are cured!" I think that's a really big struggle too; there's not a lot of people who understand what you go through.

JB: It's deeper than that and can even go back to childhood trauma. The pandemic, I feel for me and especially for other people, we peel away our layers and we say, "Oh that's it!" It's like finding a splinter in your foot, and five years have gone by and you say, "Oh, it was just a little pink, and then you keep looking at it and you realize, it went really deep."

JA: Yes, and that's what happened with me. I had things that I've gone through that I kind of always made sure I was busy. So, I didn't have to think or go through it or whatever. And then when everything shut down, I was like, "Alright, what the hell now?" That was my first experience with therapy. There was a counselor at my college. We went through everything, and she was like, "Have you ever thought about the reason why you're working and going to school and doing this and doing that is because you can't spend time with yourself? Like you can't spend that stillness thinking, and you don't know what to do with the thinking. So, by keeping busy, you're [acting] like nothing happened."

JB: Avoiding it.

JA: Yes. (Laughter) And I was like, I thought I was being productive.

I was always busy. I was dancing, working, and going to school. That was my way of coping with things and that was my way of dealing with things. I never really worked through losing my Nana because I was nine years old. Losing her at a young age and losing her that quickly was traumatic. I saw her an hour before the aneurysm ruptured and then that was it. With regards to my Papa (Jessica's grandfather), we saw him a half hour before his vitals crashed and before he was ventilated. Those two people in my life and those fatal things that happened to them happened in such a short period of time. My life changed in both instances within such a short time. I lost Papa when I was twenty-four, and I felt like I was a nine-year-old little girl all over again. I felt like I lost my Nana all over again when I lost him.

I was a young kid going through this, and now I am twenty-four, and this was something that was so similar. But even as an adult, I was very unsure how to navigate my grief and navigate my understanding of how my loved one could be alive one second and then be unresponsive. How could their life change altogether and my life change that quickly?

Even so, when I sit and think or I am asked to speak about my experience losing him or what happened in my grief journey and how I handled it and the things that I've done, I always go back to being a little kid. My coping. My way of healing. My escape. It was theater. My mom found out about a theater program in my school and threw me into it. I kicked and screamed, [but at the end of it,] I was so grateful because theater saved me. That's why things were hard for me now because I did it all throughout elementary school and middle school, high school, college. The rehearsals were late, like one o'clock in the morning. I used to take three buses home so I was like, I can't do that.

I don't really have an escape as an adult like I did as a child, and I feel like that definitely has made my grief and my depression more difficult for me. Which is crazy to think about.

JB: It's good to tap into the things that brought you joy. You're only twenty-five years old. You can go back to your joy.

JA: Which I am trying to do.

JB: Was it singing and acting, and the whole nine yards? Everything?

JA: Yes, in high school, I did musical theater. I did classical theater and was the first graduating class of my high school. So, I was part of building up the theater program; it kind of allowed me to take the weight off of my shoulders and kind of put myself and everything in a closet for a little while and become someone else.

Jessica shared her insights into how she learns best as a college student, how she set high standards for herself academically, and what this means for her mental health.

JA: I am not a big test taker. I would rather get assigned a fifteen-page paper to write than a test. I'm very big on students having a choice not only in their learning but also in how they're going to be assessed. While tests are important, I don't think that everything needs to be a test. We've gotten to the point societally, where you take a test [and when] you fail a test, you are a failure because of that grade.

School has always been my escape. I know it's unhealthy, and I'm trying to work through it. But being very transparent, I've gotten to the point where I have a 4.0. I've had it for two years now. I graduated in May, and if I get anything less than an A plus then that's on me. I feel like a failure. Because I've gone through losing my grandpa, I've gone through losing my job, you know, because of the pandemic. I've gone through being in a depression and doing school and other things. And I've made it out with the perfect score, the perfect grade. So, to me, school has always been important because that's the one thing [I have]. I didn't always have friends.

As educators, we are supposed to be there to help students, to support students. For a lot of our students, whether we know what is going on in their lives [or not], we really may be the only support system that they have. I was grateful that when I lost my Nana, I had teachers that were very supportive at a time when I bottled up everything. I came home and everyone was upset still, so I didn't want to feel like a burden. I didn't want to add on to the heartache that everyone else was going through.

School has always been that one constant in my life that nobody can take away from me. I know I'm a good student. I like reading. I like learning, doing all of those things. I speak on it from experience too. And that's something that I really want to make sure that I destigmatize in my classroom. I'm for giving students second chances when they fail a test, rather than, "Oh, you got this wrong and you got this right." What did they get wrong? What did they get right? Let's go over it. There are so many teachers that I've learned about that have placed emphasis on giving their students second, third, fourth, fifth chances. Letting them take that test over again. Allowing them to really understand what they got wrong, rather than [telling them] you got it wrong, [and] that's it.

My reason for becoming the teacher wasn't because I'm trying to breed a generation of 4.0 little minions to be perfect and get good grades and tests and everything.

My purpose is because I have gone through things in my life. Whether educators in my life have known about it [or not, I don't know]. I have had educators who have been supportive and ones who should have done more in my life. I want to be the educator I've had who picked me up when I needed it and made me feel worthy and that I could do anything and everything that I put my mind to. I want to reflect on the teachers that I had, that I needed, and weren't there for me and did things and handled situations that they should have handled differently. I want to be that support system. I understand that I have gone through things that I'm not open about. I was bullied when I was younger. My parents found out a couple years ago when I was nineteen or twenty. My mom cried. She was like, why didn't you tell us? I thought that saying something would make it worse or that it would be my fault.

JB: Have you changed during the pandemic?

JA: I feel like I have acknowledged that I need to slow down. I feel like I need to redefine myself in a way that benefits and supports my mental health.

I have acknowledged that my way of thinking for so long regarding the completion of doing things and accomplishments and everything really goes hand in hand with me being as busy as I was. And I've kind of taken on that identity of having to distract myself. But also, again, I've always thought like, I've gone through XYZ and still have the grades that I have. So, if I get anything less than that, there's no excuse because I've been through hell and back and I've done this; it's kind of me being hard on myself.

JB: Kind of? "What excuse do I have not to have that 4.0?"

JA: I feel like that has definitely played a huge role on my mental health and how I see myself and my worth that I need to attach my worth to the things that I've done and the accomplishments that I have.

JB: How do you think we're going to get out of this mental health pandemic? Because I don't know now if I see it anytime soon. I believe it has to start in the schools around things prioritizing the mental, physical, and emotional health, and not so much STEAM and STEM.

JA: I agree. I also think that what we've touched upon a little bit is the lack of resources for that, which is huge in schools to begin with, especially in college campuses and everything. I just read something yesterday that something was passed by the House to allocate more funds to more mental health resources on campuses. But like we said with the new 988 call system, they're already experiencing shortages, and they don't think they're going to have enough calls. Then on the flip side of that, a question that really hasn't been answered is who exactly is going to answer those phones, physically answer them.

JB: And are they trained properly?

JA: That too, because there's always been this conversation that if someone is going through a mental health crisis, it shouldn't just be the police [involved]. It should be, you know, trained psychologists, counselors; that's something that hasn't been addressed. So, when we get a call, is it going to be transferred to the PD? Is it going to be somebody else?

Like, what's going to happen? I definitely agree that it has to start in schools. Like everything else, we learn our ABCs in school, we learn how to multiply and divide and everything else. Wellness is something that needs more emphasis placed on it, and it should be valued more than the latter part of that is the lack of resources.

Even with New York, we have gotten rid of the bail reform. And we have people who get arrested, they go in, they see the judge, that's it, they go back out. They do the same thing again and repeat the cycle. And everybody's like, well, mental health plays a part in that because a lot of the people who are having issues with the law or have mental health issues were unable to seek care and seek treatment and everything. So, you can't have something fixed if you don't have anything to fix it. I feel like when it comes to mental health and the discussion of mental health, like I mentioned before, so many people are so quick to try to put a Band-Aid on a gaping hole. You can't do that.

JB: You're putting like a plug.

JA: And it's going to blow off. But then, the other part of that is the faculty. Teacher burnout is something that is well known, but it's not touched upon by administration, by governmental resources. It's something that's like a taboo to speak about. It's there, you know, but it's like, don't touch it because then everything is going to fall apart.

When we had our Yellow Heart Memorial, we had a professor who got up and she was hysterical. I mean, like hyperventilating, crying. My parents were with us. She grabbed my sister and hugged us and she's like, thank you so much. And she couldn't breathe, and she was like, this is the first time that my loved one has been acknowledged. And, you know, we're asking her questions. She's like, I'm the professor. I lost my father six months ago. It felt like it happened yesterday. And this is the first time that our loved ones have been acknowledged.

JA: It was so important for me to do the biweekly men's mental health virtual program that I was doing last semester with NYC Men Teach, which is a teacher's preparation program for men and minority students and cultures and neighborhoods. Because it's like, one, the stigma around mental health is very present. Men's mental health is far less spoken about. Two, on top of that, I feel being an educator when I'm going through things, I have to put all of that in my bookbag to tend to my students who need me. It's the lack of resources, but it's also the lack of funding, and it's the lack of allocation of funding, and the lack of support by those people who make these changes, who have a voice. Yes, we all have a voice, but the ones who are really in charge and making these changes, they are our voice, and as we saw yesterday, they are supposed to be the voice of the people but are the voice of the minority.

Meet Dr. Jennifer Greif Green

Associate Professor in Special Education
Boston University Wheelock College of
Education & Human Development

"It's really important that we're thinking about mental health, not just in terms of an individual, but how, as a community, to build these structures and supports in place that can bolster everybody's well-being."

—Dr. Jennifer Greif Green

I met Dr. Jennifer Greif Green when I heard about her work at Boston University, where I attended graduate school for my doctorate. We met initially and had a lot to talk about. I was so happy she agreed to be a part of this book and share her professional insights.

I asked Dr. Greif Green to share details of her work at Boston University and within schools.

Jennifer Greif Green (JG): I work at Boston University, at the Wheelock College of Education & Human Development. Mainly, I'm working with schools on trying to understand pathways into mental health services, and barriers to mental health service access for students. I'm really engaged in research around reducing inequities and access to mental health services. We know that the youth who are most likely to access mental health services are students who are white, and students who have more money, and students whose parents have completed more years of education. I'm invested in a line of research looking at how to connect students more broadly with mental health services and to reduce some of those inequities in service access.

Dr. Greif Green shared her thoughts on how we ended up in a mental health pandemic.

JG: My work is primarily with children and in schools, so I'll answer that question in the context of children and adolescents. I think, to your point, we've known for a long time that there are high rates with mental health problems among youth in the country. We know that up to about 40 percent of children and adolescents, according to some studies, will have a diagnosable mental health problem by the time they reach the age of eighteen. So, you asked how we got there. We know that a really high proportion of adults experience traumatic events in their childhood. About

60 percent of adults report having experienced an Adverse Childhood Experience (ACE), and those contribute to mental health problems that people could have experienced throughout their childhood and as they enter adulthood. And even before the pandemic, there were limited services and support available for youth. So, this is not new.

Janeane Bernstein (JB): And it's not like we were prepared for the pandemic. We didn't have pandemic training. All of a sudden, the next day, everybody's remote. I think about the impact on teachers, on administrators, and obviously students and parents.

JG: That's right. None of us knew that the pandemic was coming in the way that it was, the impact that it would have, and how long it would last. So, we had systems that were not adequately supporting youth mental health, even before the pandemic, and then those problems were exacerbated by the pandemic when this occurred.

JB: What do you think we can learn as far as how to do better in the school system? Maybe policies have to be changed? Because I see that STEM and STEAM were adopted. I don't feel that schools, across the board, have integrated mental health programming.

JG: That's right, schools have not integrated mental health programming in the same way that they have STEM and STEAM, which are great examples of subject areas that have been widely adopted and well-integrated into curricula in schools. We still, in schools, don't have routine mental health care. We don't do mental health screenings routinely in schools the same way that we do screenings for people who may need glasses, or health screenings that students receive. We don't have equivalent mental health screenings in schools. Not all schools are using social-emotional programs or universal supports for students. Almost all schools say they are underfunded and under-resourced in terms of mental health providers who can provide individual or group counseling and support for students who are in crisis or who need more intensive care.

JB: I think about what it must be like to sit in the shoes of a teacher in this pandemic. People are leaving the profession, as well as counselors.

JG: Yes, people are leaving in high rates. It's a really hard time to be a teacher and to be a counselor, and these are adults who have put themselves on the frontlines, in terms of exposure, many times to the virus. They are also trying to support students without having the resources that they need, and they have had to manage a tremendous number of shifts and changes in the last three years in terms of the structure of school. So, they need more support, and they need more resources, and they need systems, as you were saying, and policies that can support them in doing the work that they are doing so well.

JB: Through all of the conversations I've been having for this book, the seams are popping up. Even students are saying to me, "I feel that we need a better blueprint; a restructuring of what the educational model looks like, and prioritizing mental health because people aren't listening to us."

JG: I think we know that schools before the pandemic didn't work well for many of our students, were not a good fit for many of them, and weren't focused on centering equity or youth identity, or in some ways, meaningful and authentic engagement with material. And that's become even more clear to us in the past few years, and we hear youth in my work who say that they liked it more when they were remote, and they felt like the things that they were doing during remote learning were more meaningful. They felt more connected to their family, and they liked that experience more. I think that's a sign to us, as we're thinking about what education and what schools should look like going forward, that can more broadly meet the needs of children and adolescents, that what we were doing before just didn't work for everybody.

JB: I can see why students would feel safer remotely than they do in person. Perhaps they can't be their authentic selves and they don't feel that they can be open about their mental health needs.

JG: I think that's true for some students, and I have heard that from families of children with anxiety, in particular, that anxiety in some children dropped when they were engaged in school remotely. Obviously, that wasn't true for everybody. For many children, anxiety went way up during the pandemic, but I think that this gives us a chance to really think about how to individualize what we're doing and recognize the obvious: that different children need different things and different structures around them to support them.

JB: When I see all these things in the news, practically every day—Mental Health America posting something, the Attorney General came out with a paper—I was thinking, "Okay, this is very important, I'm glad that we're talking about it. What are we doing about it? And it can't be in a few years from now; what are we doing about it now?"

JG: Right. I'm optimistic that talking about it is doing something. That all of a sudden there is more discussion in the media and more discussion among adults about mental health. The optimistic side of me believes that will make a difference because so many of the reasons that children don't receive mental health services are related to stigma and fear of what will happen if they reach out for help. But you're right, we need to be doing more. We need to be thinking more about what we can be doing broadly to support the youth. I think the increase in access to mental health services through Telehealth is an important step. I'll be really curious to see what happens with Telehealth moving forward and ways it can help to increase access to care for families, especially [those] that are living in harder to reach places and who haven't traditionally had as easy access to mental health services as people in Boston or around LA do.

JB: I think we talked about this another time, but I feel that if we set up some preventative models and some preventative education, perhaps the strain will be less on the teachers and the counselors, and students can come together on issues that are not huge, to kind of deescalate. And they can share, and they can be more open about what's on their mind.

JG: Yes, you're saying a lot of students can talk to each other and can provide support to each other if they know how to do that, and if we as adults can help facilitate these kinds of conversations.

JB: Do you have any thoughts on how—this is a really challenging time—we can see this as a way to create positive change?

JG: I do think that talking more about mental health is really important. We talk a lot more about physical health still, especially now, than about mental health. We have routine screenings for physical health problems, we have routine care for physical health; we don't have systems that are the same for mental health, and we don't talk about it in the same way. If someone said to me or said to you that at some point in their lifetime most children would have a physical health problem, we'd say, "Of course they will, that makes sense." People have colds, people have the flu. Even before COVID-19, people had physical health problems. The fact that we see mental health problems so differently, I think, is a sign that there are some opportunities to shift our thinking and to recognize that most people will have a mental health problem in their lifetime or be closely connected to someone who does. It's not about other people, it's about us and people who are close to us. I think that those shifts in thinking can change how we think about embedding mental health supports into schools and communities in new ways.

JB: I don't know if you can answer this. How do policies change? Let's say somebody creates this model in the Boston school system, and we want to share it across the country. How do we create positive change about mental health?

JG: I think one way to do that is to make sure that we're looking at data to show what works. Sometimes policies are put into place, and no one ever evaluates them or looks at them or has some way of knowing, first, whether they work at all, and second, for whom they work best. So, having funding structures in place to look at those data to see what's working, and then to link that to important outcomes. So for schools, that can be grades, graduation rates, attendance rates. All those things are really important for schools. So, the more we can link our mental health resources and supports to those key outcomes, those metrics that school evaluations are based on for changing policy—and similarly, if we can link data on mental health services to reductions in other costs, and reductions in healthcare costs—those become powerful points for bringing forward to legislators and policymakers.

JB: Because I do feel this is an extraordinary time to really connect with students and to find out what their needs are, and to test out ideas that could possibly help across the country. As I said when we started this conversation, we adopted STEM and STEAM, it's really time to do something about mental health.

JG: I agree. I think this is a really important time to be thinking about how to grab onto these opportunities and to move forward.

JB: One of the things that came up for me months ago—I was talking with a psychiatrist from another university, and he said, "You know, a student can get a full scholarship to a prestigious university and have to sleep in their car and go to the food bank. And they can't travel to go see their family because they have no money." There are so many issues that impact students. It's really important to consider that.

JG: Yeah, and in thinking about your questions about what's happened during the pandemic—the extent of loss, and food insecurity, and job loss is really important to consider when we're thinking about mental health as well.

JB: I know, two weeks ago, I saw an article how there's a lot of abuse going on at home. And I think, "Okay, well why is that happening?" Could be a mental health issue. Could be stress of parents; they lost income, they split up. People have passed away. There are so many things you could fill in the blank on.

JG: Yes, so, in my work I think a lot about how teachers can be people who identify students who need support, and how teachers make decisions around whether and how to refer students for support. So, for example, if a teacher sees a student with their head down on a desk, how does the teacher decide about what might be happening with that student, and whether or not to connect them with supports. And if they do connect them with support, they need to decide if they're going to send that student to the school counselor, or psychologist, or to the school nurse, or to the principal's office. There are these different pathways that students can end up on, depending on how teachers make those decisions. I've been spending a lot of time talking with teachers and thinking a lot about what kinds of preparation and support teachers need in order to recognize what might be a mental health problem, and to make decisions about referrals that will be supportive of students, and hopefully lead to them to being more like to be connected with services and not disciplinary routes in particular.

JB: Right, because it could be anything. It could be the kid didn't sleep last night. Or they are suffering with a mental health issue. There are so many factors. So, it sounds like it's a training issue that has to happen for teachers?

JG: I think a lot of it is a training issue. We know that teachers make these decisions based on their mental health literacy. The idea of mental health literacy is that each person has a background or a store of knowledge and attitudes and beliefs about mental health. So, teachers enter these situations with their own extent of knowledge about mental health and attitudes about mental health and mental health services. Coupled with the context they're a part of mental health literacy informs the decisions they make.

JB: And now, in 2022, the world is more complex.

JG: It sure is.

JB: They're trying to meet their education goals, and their deadlines, and everything else. Do you feel like we need to have less of a focus on grades and scores and more on mental health and wellness? Because really, long term, I think that to me, that's what matters most.

JG: I'm on the same page as you. I think that's what matters most, too. I'm not convinced that grades and scores are great indicators of meaningful learning experiences for youth, in general.

JB: I've been saying to students, "If you are having a tough time right now, cut yourself some slack. This is not going to predict your future." And I say this from my own personal story from having to leave my mom at sixteen; she was not mentally well. I had to go live with my dad. This was right before finals. I was, I would say, a D/F student. And my ACES score was very high, and I didn't discover that until recently. So, the point is, you're going to go through all kinds of ups and downs. It's okay. Really, it's not going to predict your future.

JG: I think that's a great message to give to students—that regardless of what has happened to them before that they can make decisions moving forward that will determine the course of where they go as an adult and in the future.

JB: When I came to Boston years ago, I had lost my job in less than a year, and it wasn't because of something I had done. The economy had taken a dive. I thought, "Oh no, what do I do now? I don't know anyone." It didn't help that I had a break-up around the same time. So, it just felt like everything was crumbling. A while later I decided to go back to grad school, which is why I went to BU, because I felt I wasn't happy in my career, and I wanted to do something very meaningful. I remember talking with my dad and he said, "Why don't you take two classes?" One was that qualitative research class, which changed everything.

JG: Well, we were lucky to get you here, and I think sometimes it's those small steps that start to shape someone's path in a different way.

JB: Anything else you'd like to add?

JG: I think just that if the last year has taught us anything, one of the things that I think has been showing clearly is that who we are and what we do impacts whole communities. Decisions that we make don't just impact ourselves but impact communities broadly. We can think about mental health the same way: how we care for our own mental health and the mental health of our children and our families can have a dramatic impact on those around us. To go back to teachers, we see that when teachers have a higher well-being and are feeling better in their classrooms, their students do better. So, it's really important that we're thinking about mental health, not just in terms of an individual, but how, as a community, to build these structures and supports in place that can bolster everybody's well-being.

JB: One last thing I'll add to that is, a lot of people are saying—all different ages—it's a time to really be kinder, more empathetic, and compassionate.

JG: Yes, all times would be good for that.

Meet Octavio Hernandez

Middle School Teacher, School Board Member – Florida

"Mental health—right now the only way out (of the pandemic) is parents understanding it's okay to seek help. I think parents understanding that mental health is a real thing and supporting children to have someone to talk to."

—Octavio Hernandez

I read about Octavio Hernandez in the *New York Times* when he spoke passionately about student mental health and gun control. We met one Saturday morning by phone and had a very long and meaningful conversation about life as a teacher, the debate about gun control, and the changes he would like to see moving forward.

Octavio Hernandez (OH): My biggest concern, of course, is where I live; this is a very pro-gun area. "Teachers should carry (guns)." They don't even trust us with books. The books get banned. Our superintendent had to pull eighteen books, and they had to get overlooked just because there was a group of parents that got together and said that these books are inappropriate for high schoolers. Some people are asking that our teachers carry and you're yearning for more problems, and you're fixating on solving a symptom, not the actual cause. What keeps happening is we keep putting Band-Aids instead of healing the actual disease.

They don't understand what we're going through right now. We literally had this conversation with our fellow teachers. More and more teachers quit. We have to carry more of the load, more students, bigger classes, and we're going to come to the point where we can actually teach. What I mean by "just teach"—to me, teaching more than just a subject area.

We're pillars in the community of education, of society. I hope the parents trust us to guide the kids in doing the right thing for themselves; this is what it's supposed to be, and when you start adding something as dangerous as "Where's my gun?" in the classroom, I start to get upset. I get angry because they can't trust us with books, and it infuriates me. If I wanted to become a police officer, I would have become a police officer, but I wanted to teach. I shouldn't have to defend myself in a school.

Where children cope with the safest place it (school) is supposed to be, I'm actually supposed to be the most frightened to be at; it is supposed to be the safest environment for our students, for their minds, for the well-being, for their social skills. Now it has become the most dangerous place for them to be outside of driving in the car; it happens so often that now people are just like, "Well, let's do something to protect ourselves rather do something about guns." Let's do something about mental health because obviously there are some mental health issues.

Octavio mentioned how students and parents are experiencing numerous stress and strain leading to mental health issues. I shared the thoughts that went through my mind when I heard about the shooting in Uvalde, Texas, wondering about the backstory of the shooter, his homelife and relationship with his parents. Yes, we have a gun issue, but it's deeply rooted in mental health. Here's how he responded.

Octavio: The mental health part is going to get even worse in my opinion. I see it. These last two years, there's a cloud over the classroom. These kids are foggy. What's going on? There are supposed to be answers for them. Even we don't have answers to what's going on. There is war, epidemic, civil disobedience everywhere. Kids are going through this, and parents are going through crisis, and I can't imagine seeing a kid and seeing his parents have mental health issues, right? And it's coming up more and more. Children look up to their parents, and they're supposed to have all the answers, and when you look at your parents, you see they're as messed up as you are.

I believe the mentality of the American dream of working for everything that you want. People don't realize that you mostly have to sacrifice a lot of things you love to achieve your goals. And that in itself makes us alienate ourselves. But now you add a new way of communicating—social media. You're also disconnecting, so we're telling you to be successful, and you have to disconnect. You have to work hard and make that a priority, but if we disconnect from our friends, what is the purpose? I think you're right. We were already in a crisis mentally before because of the way our system was made.

Insights in the pandemic:

OH: What are we trying to prove? Because if we have trauma in our childhood, and now we're adults, and we feel like we just have to go, go, go, and we're trying to prove something and we keep ourselves busy, right? Everybody started realizing, what's the purpose of my life?

Why am I here? Like, oh my God, I've been working, working, working. That's why you see this giant migration of people from San Francisco, Dallas, New York. They're all moving down to Florida because it's cheaper; that's where the money is. And they worked so hard, and they're like, I'm done. We saw so many people die from COVID. No matter how much money you had. It didn't matter if you're sick. At the beginning of COVID, you had to be somebody really, really important to get good treatment. So that made a lot of people question their life. "Am I happily married? Am I happy being a stay-at-home mom?" I think that's what happened.

Octavio was featured on CNN and shared the controversy behind teachers and Socio-Emotional Learning (SEL). He feels strongly that SEL is needed right now.

OH: We hear social and emotional learning—that's what they're trying to get rid of. And that's what got me on a CNN interview. What are you trying to get rid of? No, that's what we're trying to *do*—social-emotional learning. They were saying that teachers are telling students how to be in touch with their feelings. It's about knowing how to control those emotions. The next generation of sixth graders, middle schoolers, because they missed fourth and fifth grade, have actual structure milestones, and they're going into middle school with no foundation of a social filter on behaving.

Everybody's starting to accept that mental health is just as important as physical health. I tell my students about seeing a therapist and seeing a counselor. I tell them, I see somebody to talk to somebody; it's not even about you being mentally broken. I tell my students if I were to go into any kind of working field right now it would be engineering, medical, or counseling, mental health counseling.

I asked them if someone broke their leg, would you be upset that they went to a doctor? Would you make fun of me for seeing a doctor for a broken leg? No. So why would you make fun of anyone because of counseling? They're going through something traumatic. And when I say that, then they all like, maybe they saw their parents in the hospital for a month. Or maybe they've seen their parents get divorced. Their grandma passed away or brothers and sisters were sick and everybody's just like, "Okay, yeah. It's okay to talk to them." I bring it up every class. I bring up all my meetings. And you're right, this should be talked about more.

Janeane Bernstein (JB): I feel that there needs to be some changes now—not in a few years—in how schools teach about mental health and how this is prioritized because, yes, you can push them to do well and get into a great college. But if they're not mentally strong and skilled in self-care, what happens when they go to college?

OH: You're absolutely right. The first time I taught middle school, I had the honors kids, but they also gave me the kids that have behavioral problems because they know I get along. I tried to connect with all age groups, all social status children, but my honor kids, I push them and then I tell them you need to know when to shut it down. If you're mentally exhausted, shut it off. Because you're talking about mental health and how to promote it, and the problem we have with mental health is a lot of people think that it's against capitalism or against us self-fulfilling. You don't need to be successful in everything. Just be human. Enjoy life sometimes. I think it goes against our values. We're fighting for mental health now to be introduced in the classroom.

I called my mother, and she was the first one I told, "Hey, I'm going to get separated." And she's like, "You're sure?" I'm like I can't do it. I don't want my kids to see this. This is not healthy. This is not what "married" looks like.

She said, "Okay, you need to take care of yourself first." That's the first thing she said to me, and I broke down crying. Because I told her I don't know what that means.

What does that mean, "self-care"? Because every time I try to do something for myself, I feel guilty.

JB: Really?

OH: Oh my god. Absolutely. I mean, like it's selfish.

Octavio talked about his struggles growing up and how his backstory shaped who he is today.

OH: I skipped two grades. I graduated two years younger than all my friends. Now I'm getting older, and I'm telling my story to other adults who are like, "This is not real. How are you normal?" But I feel like those trials and tribulations are what have allowed me to be a matter of fact because I've gone through them, and I survived them being outspoken. I don't want that to happen to anyone else. I don't want my reason I became a teacher part of it. Not one teacher ever pulled me aside because I used to pass tests like nothing; I was just a troublemaker. I try to mentor kids in many different ways. I will show you a lot of the letters they write me I have in my room, and they tell me things like that. You know, "Thank you for pushing me. Thank you for mentoring me. Thank you for being supportive."

JB: You instill a love of learning, which is key and a growth mindset; they will take that with them forever. You're opening their eyes up to other things and outside of your classroom, they're still thinking of you. How do you see we're going to get out of this mental health pandemic?

OH: It's either going to collapse and then we're finally going to do something about it. A lot of teachers from all over are at that point where if you ask us to carry guns, I think it's going to be a big problem. I tell my teachers right now we're the ones that made it through. We're the ones who are sticking out the pandemic. I think once we get the communities involved on a local level that's when parent involvement and class sizes, in my opinion, are the biggest things to education.

I honestly think that the way to get out it is either going to be a mental collapse and maybe talk about the school industry. I'm in Polk County. My school is the largest employer of teachers. They're the largest employer education system. People think we're just replaceable. We're not. Nobody wants to do this for $47,000 a year. You really got to have a love for it. And then once you get in, you realize that it's a skeleton crew. You're not going to be able to sustain working there.

When I got divorced, first thing [I did was] I took my kids to therapy. You need to talk to someone that's not in the middle, someone objective. The first time, they hated it, but when they [left the sessions], they felt good. They can do it throughout their lifetime; it's needed. I try to teach my kids the way I wish my parents would have taught me. I'm very open with them. It doesn't matter what religion or race you are or politics you follow, mental health affects all of us.

Meet Ross Gothelf

11th Grade Civics and Economics Teacher – Denver, Colorado

"I think everyone has just become numb. I think back to the day of the shooting in Texas and my immediate reaction, because I saw it when I was at school, was nothing. I had no reaction at first because it was like I needed to get through my day. I needed to teach; I couldn't process it immediately. When I was able to finally sit down and process, I read something on Twitter by Clint Smith III, and he said these kids ate their favorite cereals

this morning, played with their friends on the bus, thought about summer break, and now twenty of them had their beds empty tonight. That really hit home."

—Ross Gothelf

I met Ross through his sister, Mallory Gothelf, who is also included in this book and on my series. Ross has been a teacher for over nine years and shared what life has been like as an educator in the pandemic, what changes he would like to see in education and society, and his thoughts on becoming better humans.

Ross Gothelf (RG): We got out March 13, 2020. The years 2020 to 2021 were completely online for us here in Denver and a huge adjustment. Coming back into this most recent school year, we thought "This will be great. We're back in person." Little did we realize what we were in for. This has been the most difficult school year since I started teaching back in 2013.

Janeane Bernstein (JB): Why is that?

RG: I think the return to in-person learning. During the pandemic, everybody was talking about how we needed to reinvent education, revolutionize what we're doing, and we can't go back to the way things were before. But then when everyone got back, I think everyone was so excited to be back in person that we just wanted to resume, kind of like we see it all other aspects of life. People just want to go back to the way things were, but there is no way.

JB: There has been so much pressure on teachers and counselors and having to deal with the pandemic, but at a policy level there needs to be preventative initiatives, peer-to-peer, etc. When I talk to some schools, they'll say we have "mental health week," and I feel there needs to be better training and education to prioritize mental health because once they leave K–12, if their mental health is not in check, where does that leave them in college? And then into adulthood?

RG: I completely agree. I think about what does it take for human beings to be successful in general, right? As a society, we spend tons of money on our physical well-being, apparel, gym memberships, diets, and all that stuff, but we pay little attention to our mental being. I work in a school that's overwhelmingly students of color, Black and Brown students. The overwhelming majority also have free and reduced lunch, and so you think about the stressors that growing up in poverty places on you, along with various other systems of oppression that are working against students that I work with. Mental health has to be at the front and center of everything that we do. But I think that I agree that a lot of it gets kind of watered down or we have a social worker on it. But she's so overworked that she's not able to really see everyone and every time. We have a school psychologist, but she's only there a couple of days because we share with another campus. We need more focus on mental health to be able to do the things that we would like to do.

Mental health plays a big part at the school level. I think a lot of people who are in positions of power, they're making decisions about funding for schools. In Colorado, we've historically been very low in terms of per pupil funding. There's a lot of like perfect budget maneuvers that have been kind of implemented to keep education from getting the funding that they should be receiving, but even go to the national level. Politicians' children will be okay, they'll get access to the private therapies that they need, that everybody needs and deserves access to, right. But they are able to turn a blind eye to those who don't have those opportunities. And they'll say, "Oh, we'll throw more money at it" without taking a look at whether this is delivering the outcomes that we intended for this money to achieve. It's such a big issue that it's hard to really begin pointing the finger at "Hey, we need to start here!" But a common understanding and agreement is a good place to start.

JB: We have to start somewhere. The students I've been talking to are saying things like, "I don't feel heard. I don't feel like I can talk to somebody. I'm not going to talk to that one guidance counselor. I don't feel they really get me. I'd rather go talk to my peers." They don't feel a sense of connection and compassion. I'm not saying that's at every school, but it's for a lot of students.

RG: I completely agree. As an educator, my first task before I can even instruct anybody is to build relationships with young people. If people don't think you care about them, they are not going to listen to anything you say. I've had a number of kids tell me some quite horrific things this year. That's always been the case that kids will confide in me. The incidence rates this year is higher than had been previously, and it just points to how badly people are hurting right now. A lot of it deals with people not having the material resources they need, and other issues get compounded.

There needs to be opportunities for students to connect with one another, validate each other's experiences and also opportunities for hope. That is even difficult for adults. If I was a sixteen or seventeen-year-old right now and I look at the climate crisis, issues around homelessness, housing in Denver, the war in Ukraine, and whatever existential issue you want to point to, it seems to be coalescing right in this moment. There needs to be greater attention paid to mental health and instilling hope. I identify as a millennial. I think my generation and the generation above me didn't do a great job of working together. There's a lot of conflict among us. Gen Z and the millennials and whoever else need to get together and start figuring things out. The time for haggling is over; I think Gen Z really does understand that.

JB: I am so impressed with a lot of people in the Gen Z demographic in that they are very open about issues that have not been discussed. They'll say, I'm taking a mental health day. I need to focus on my mental health. They stand up for things that are so important, whether it's people experiencing homelessness, climate change, diversity, and inclusion, and so on. These are such important issues. As they become adults, they're going to prioritize these issues where there's been apathy.

RG: I tell my students, and I think they probably think I'm being corny, but they give me a lot of hope for the future. Don't get me wrong, there's a lot of work that needs to be done. When I see things, they're willing to persevere through; it's more than just survive. They do some pretty phenomenal things. I think about a student of mine, and she's not unique in this situation, but within the past couple years, her dad was deported. Now, she is one of our top achieving students and is a national Speech and Debate qualifier and was number one in the country. I think about that. That gives me a lot of hope. Young people are spectacular, and sometimes we just need to create the conditions to allow them to thrive and step back and let them do their thing.

JB: When you talk about hope, which is so important, we need to build positivity, and when we give them opportunities to do something that is purpose-driven and meaningful, and perhaps takes them out of that mindset of whatever it is they're dealing with, they're shifting and helping someone that is experiencing homelessness or whatever, fill in the blank. That's going to lift them up; it's going to change their perspective.

RG: Agree 100 percent. We've had students who will be exposed to an internship, or a guest speaker and they connect with that speaker, and all of a sudden, a whole new world opens up before them. I think that's part of our job in education is to be connected, particularly in communities where those social networks or access to services is not part and parcel of your household. Opportunities are great, but we need to, as a society, go back to what we said before. There's a lot we can do to create better access, so that people will not only get exposed to those opportunities but really are able to see them through. I have a ton of students who cannot do a summer program because there's a cost and travel fee and they need to work to help their parents out. Until we're able to do that, I don't think we're really creating equitable access for everyone.

JB: You're right. And that's such a letdown—to be excited about an opportunity but to not have the financial means to get on that plane or for your room and board; that could change their trajectory if they have that opportunity.

RG: Or here's this great internship but it's unpaid. I think employers, whether private or public sector—I think there has been movement to provide scholarships. You never really know how much is actually being offered, right? I'll leave it there.

I shared with Ross how recently I spoke to students about "the keys to success" and how success is probably not what they think or what they were told to believe. Success is facing life's challenges, the disappointments, rejections, and losses and picking yourself up each time with grace and strength, not bitterness and deep-rooted sadness. Life will continue to be bumpy, and when you learn to have grit, and introspection, you can face situations with a resilient mindset. For example, say to yourself, "Yes, I failed. I got rejected. I was broken up with, I was _____, but I am going to keep on going, take really great care of me, and nurture myself through this situation, and each time I will become better and stronger at handling what comes my way."

Ross continued by talking about academic expectations and the fine line between balancing empathy with expectations and requirements.

RG: I would say you need to add high expectations. That's a tough line to balance, particularly coming out of the pandemic or the current iteration of the pandemic—this idea that yes, students have been through a lot. We can't keep saying that "It's okay," you're going through a lot. It's not okay to be late to class over and over; it's not okay to not put forth your best effort. And so, it's tough. You really feel for a kid telling you that dad just walked out last night. I want to create space for you. Let's talk if you want to talk. I hope you have an adult in the building who you can trust and talk to but also, you're seventeen years old. I need you to do this assignment. I can give you more time. We're still going to need to get things done; it's a tough balance though because sometimes your heart just breaks for these young people. And you're also like, I'm not their parent. That's not my role to play. I can't fix society. As much as I would love to fix it in this moment, I can't, all of a sudden, double the staff at Denver Health so that there's a therapist who can see you sooner than a month.

Our school has a social justice focus, and we always try and focus on how we are seeing race and class, gender, and sexuality. How are we seeing those issues intersect in our given context? Dena Simmons, who is in the mental health sphere, talks about social emotional learning, and we can't just do it without talking about race when we are instructing Black and Brown students. There's a reason why conditions for our students who are Black and Brown in particular are the way that they are. If we don't teach them the history of how we've gotten to where we are as a society, then we're doing them a disservice. We're just perpetuating this idea that you as an individual should just overcome the obstacles that have been put in front of you.

Ross shared his concerns about public education and why teachers are leaving their profession.

RG: As a society, we're not going to fix all of our ills by focusing on education, but we would solve a large number of them if we were able to do public education right. I'm not trying to be an alarmist or exaggerate, but I really feel like we're in a moment where public education is on the precipice of no longer existing. I know that sounds crazy to say, but I saw a statistic earlier this year at the Colorado Educators Association, which is a statewide union organizing body. They said that in a survey, two out of three teachers in Colorado were thinking about not returning next year. That's already on the high number of vacancies nationwide.

In some states, teachers have to work two to three jobs. Let's start paying teachers more.

JB: And valuing them.

RG: And valuing them. How do we value someone in our capitalist society? It is either by compensating them more or giving them more time to do the things that they need to do. Those are really the only two ways you can compensate someone. Unless we start doing that, I'm worried. We talked about hope, but from a system level, I'm very concerned about where things will go in public education. And what really makes it scary for me is knowing who will be worse off as a result, which is our students in low-income communities, recently arrived immigrants, Black and Brown indigenous students—that's what keeps me up at night.

JB: Have you known a lot of teachers who have left the profession?

RG: Yes. Just at my school alone off the top of my head, I would say at least five staff members resigned throughout the year. Our principal resigned as well. Good luck finding a good chemistry teacher to begin with, but then trying to replace one mid-year. Our tenth graders probably had three core content area teachers leave throughout the year, and then behaviors were horrible because there were no expectations. There are no systems in place, and compounding that is the fact that the last time they were in the school, they were in eighth grade. What makes it difficult is because talking to one of those people who resigned, knowing the reason they resigned, I don't blame them.

But from a "Hey, I work at this school" level, it sucks because you're like, now, I'm going to have to give up an off period to sub more often. We sub in-house when we can't find subs. Frankly, a lot of people are just fed up with being treated poorly by the school system, and now society is suddenly villainizing teachers for speaking truth to power, and it's alarming.

JB: It's very alarming, and with regards to all the shootings, it seems like every day there's another shooting. Why do you think that is, and what can be done about it?

RG: At a fundamental level, if people didn't have guns, then this wouldn't be an issue. I taught for two years in Madrid, Spain. And in my two years there not once did I ever have to worry about getting shot on the street or in a school because guns aren't a thing. Unfortunately, Pandora's box has been opened, and I know people from all sides have their own perspectives, but it's just too easy to get a gun in our society. Yes, people make the argument, "There's plenty of people that own these guns that don't go shoot up schools, movie theaters, or grocery stores. But they're still able to get these guns. There needs to be serious action taken on guns.

I am not saying that no one should have a gun. I know that there's a lot of arguments that the issue goes beyond just guns. There's violence ingrained in U.S. society because of what the U.S. has been. People don't feel safe right now. I have colleagues who don't feel safe. Further compounding that is this sense of hopelessness, because we talk about these shootings for a couple of days, and then we go on to the next one. I told this to a colleague recently, Janeane. It was somewhat in jest, but I think this whole year has kind of been "Let's laugh to keep from crying." I told a colleague, "Hey, if I die in a school shooting—if there's a shooting at my school, I'm going to put my body on the line. That's my promise to these students' families; their child is going to be safe while they're with me—put my body outside Mitch McConnell's office wherever the Senate Majority Leader is for the Republicans." We're at a point where we can't continue this. How many mass shootings need to have taken place since Uvalde for someone to finally say enough is enough?

I think it's going to take something like a general strike, where as a society people say we can't continue. We can't continue. I teach civics. The system is not set up. We can claim we live in a democracy, but the reality is that we don't. We don't live in a democracy. I would love to live in one. That's not the reality because the reality is that we have a minority of senators who have a disproportionate amount of power over what can be done in this country, and that doesn't align with the views of the majority of folks on a number of issues.

JB: There's so much mental duress right now. It's really concerning. I think about the levels of anxiety that have risen because of all these events, and all this information is so accessible on social media.

RG: Social media has been great. It can also be quite toxic. Instagram's own internal research spoke to that before it was buried by the powers that be at Facebook or Meta. We shouldn't be surprised that things are as bad as they are right now. You talked about how millions of people lost their jobs during the pandemic. We lost over a million people, which is a number that's hard to process. You think about one individual—losing someone's Mom. That's huge. A tragedy in its own right. We have all these problems already—being exploited or not doing well to begin with. Now people are like why is the crime rate going up, why are mass shootings happening, why are schools struggling so badly? It shouldn't be surprising, and as you continue to harp on mental health, we have answers. They are not going to be the one antidote to all of society's problems. We've got to start somewhere.

Ross feels optimistic about the road ahead for Gen Z and sees their potential in shaping the future.

RG: I tend to start heading in a more hopeful direction. For the reasons we discussed before, this group of young people will have to be our greatest generation. I think that they can very well live up to that potential if we allow them to.

I appreciate the work you're doing to continue to highlight the need for greater connection among young people in particular, just the call to action on mental health. More people need to be having these conversations. The fact that we're able to have this conversation gives me hope that there's a lot of good happening already and that we can continue to push for more in the days ahead.

* * *

Now, take a moment to consider what life must be like for teachers in Ukraine living in a time of war. The closest I came to this was a conversation with the co-chair of EdCamp Ukraine, who shared what life is like for himself, his family, and the forty thousand teachers who are part of EdCamp Ukraine. Little did he know that such a purpose-driven, impactful organization would be the glue to keep teachers connected and hopeful in a time of daily uncertainty and trauma. While the U.S. is reeling from COVID-19, people in Ukraine have a war to contend with and the daily sounds of alarms reverberating throughout the day. There are no plans being made.

There is only today and living in the now because life in Ukraine is fractured and uncertain.

Meet Dr. Oleksandr Elkin

Inspirer of the EdCamp movement in Ukraine

"You will not find a Ukrainian who is not under stress, traumatized, or even experienced PTSD. It's a huge challenge. Therefore, I salute the decision of the First Lady of Ukraine, Olena Zelenska, to make mental health programs her priority, supporting Ukrainians and helping people overcome all these challenges."

—Dr. Oleksandr Elkin

Dr. Oleksandr Elkin is a Ukrainian public figure and the founder of the responsible teaching movement, EdCamp Ukraine, a forty-thousand-strong community of teachers who engage in personal, professional, and systematic change in their educational institutions. He is also chairman of the board of the non-governmental organization of the same name, EdCamp Ukraine. I met Oleksandr through Elaine Miller-Karas, the co-founder and director of Innovation, Vision, and Creativity for the Trauma Resource Institute. A special thank you to Dr. Bryan Robinson and Elaine for introducing me to Oleksandr. After my initial meeting with Oleksandr, I recalled a conversation with my beloved grandmother, Madeline. When I was fifteen years old, she made sure I learned how to pronounce my great-grandmother's maiden name—Minnie Malishkevich. A deep dive into Google led me to discover that both Minnie and her husband Nathan (my great-grandfather) were from Kyiv, Ukraine.

I met Oleksandr prior to this interview, and we spoke for a while. Hearing about his family and life in Ukraine was very emotional for me, and I was struck by his strength and drive to create resilience not only in his own life but in the lives of thousands of teachers who are part of EdCamp Ukraine. I began our conversation by asking Oleksandr to describe what life is like for him right now in Ukraine in the midst of a war with Russia.

Oleksandr Elkin (OE): My wife and I have a deal. It's about analyzing the experience we are going through now as a family, thinking about right after the victory of Ukraine and coming back to understanding what has happened to our country and to ourselves within these unparalleled war circumstances. What I can say about the current state is that this is a new challenging chapter in the history of Ukraine, its people, and the world generally. We can't bring back the past. I mean, the past before February 24, when the massive invasion started, and we can't predict the future. I should say a future. The only thing, and this is my biggest personal lesson—that the war teaches me—is to stay in the current moment, to value and celebrate every day. For instance, yesterday was the thirty-first anniversary of our country, our Independence Day.

I calculated in a security app the sirens we had, the alarms. It gives prompts when Russia is bombing Ukraine or the particular region you're in. I calculated that in Kyiv, where we stay now as IDPs (internally displaced persons forced to leave)—we are from Kharkiv—there were eight alarms on that day.

Janeane Bernstein (JB): One day? Eight alarms!

OE: Yes. So, you can't predict it. You can't control it. And this was the toughest thing for me. I overslept at the beginning of the war. I woke up at 8:00 a.m. when my wife cried, "The war started!" The first bombing of Kharkiv was around 5:00 a.m. I remember that feeling in your body, in your thoughts, that your life is broken. It's because you can't plan, you know? I'm a very organized, aim-oriented person. I had plans for years ahead and that feeling that I couldn't plan (pause) a month—no—even a day ahead. An hour ahead. And this is something that symbolizes this experience for me, and the lesson is not to recollect the past. Don't think too much about the future. Try to stay in the moment, and this is what supports me a lot.

JB: This is a very important lesson. Please tell me about EdCamp Ukraine, how you got involved in this teaching initiative.

OE: I have a wonderful quote, which I use when I share a story about EdCamp. Surprisingly, I got a present with this quote. It's a special bookmark, and these are the words of Margaret Mead, a famous anthropologist: "Never doubt that a small group of thoughtful committed citizens can change the world. Indeed, it's the only thing that ever has." The EdCamp idea, I believe, is an excellent demonstration of what Margaret is saying to us in this piece of wisdom because it originated as an idea of eleven educators who met together in Philadelphia in 2010 to think about what they could do to change how teachers receive professional development.

In many countries of the world and even in progressive educational systems, this remains a challenge. So, people with a degree in education go to school, and they frequently freeze in their development, unfortunately. The massive challenge for the States, Ukraine, and many other countries is that people are quitting the teaching profession. You have enthusiasm while you develop in the lifelong learning process, and the EdCamp idea is simple yet effective because of the innovative approach to professional growth. The format of EdCamp is peer-to-peer; it's not when an expert enters the room and tells you what to do and what to follow. It's like a conversation of practitioners, very horizontal, based on sharing, where there is no one, precise, correct answer to the challenge, like in life. Complex issues don't have one answer.

A lot of things depend on the context. And this is why EdCamp became so powerful. It is spread in every state of your country, but it has roots in forty-five more countries. The EdCamp community is the second largest after the United States family. I founded EdCamp when I stepped off from a career in IT, and it was also connected to the war. The war in Ukraine, this Russia invasion, started not this February. It started at least in 2014, when they occupied Crimea, when they occupied parts of Donetsk and Luhansk regions. Some historians think that the war started even hundreds of years before, so it has been a long war. Personally, I felt it in 2014 with the Revolution of Dignity; it was shocking and a very transformative experience for a lot of Ukrainians. I got this feeling, "Now or never." I decided to bring the EdCamp idea here because, in my background, I was always connected to education—to the EdTech business and higher education institutions. I felt from my previous experience that no innovations could blossom if educators were not ready for them. Because people are the ones heading the process, not technology and not physical environments. People are at the center of a solution. In 2014, we started preparing for the first EdCamp event in Ukraine. Nobody believed that teachers would be willing to share in an open manner in Ukraine.

In 2015, we conducted the first event, which gathered 325 participants.

JB: That's great.

OE: Not much.

JB: It's something.

OE: But something, and that was, I think, the most touching event from everywhere we organized. From that moment, we facilitated over 250 events of different sizes.

JB: Wow!

OE: And so now we have a community of forty thousand like-minded educators from every second school in Ukraine who are bonded with this feeling of changing our secondary school education for the better and who co-created the new Ukrainian school reform of competencies for life; this is one of the most supported reforms in Ukraine. Sometimes, I think that maybe these seven years from foundation to the current day were to help us survive in this war because our educators in Ukraine are heroes. (You can feel their spirit in the interview series "My war: The lessons for Ukraine and Humanity," https://www.edcamp.ua/en/my-war-lessons-en/)

JB: Absolutely. You know, I have chills right now. Because as you started to say, I believe that seven years was a way of preparing for this moment. I was thinking the same thing because look at the sense of connection and empowerment, and you are valuing these teachers and look at what they have to deal with right now. If there wasn't an EdCamp Ukraine, where would they be? You have given educators such a sense of meaning, purpose, and connection, which is everything for mental health. Because if they don't feel valued and mentally strong, how are they going to do this essential work they are doing?

OE: It's how the law of interconnectedness works. This is, by the way, among the core ideas of the Social, Emotional, and Ethical learning program, which we are implementing nationally after meeting with His Holiness Dalai Lama, Elaine Miller-Karas, and Emory University colleagues in 2019. So yes, you're right. Our educators are continuing to do their professional duties, conducting classes from the underground and shelters under bombing and shelling, and being evacuated sometimes in very hard conditions, but this is not the only kind of their contribution. They are also supporting their communities. They are leaders in the *hromadas* (the Ukrainian word for "communities"). They are responsible citizens, and they support the territorial defense and the army. They're volunteering and helping IDPs. For instance, my family was able to survive only due to the help of EdCampers. When we were escaping from Kharkiv and the bombing, we were sharing a car, and there was no food, no petrol, there was no place where you could stay because everything was overbooked, and you couldn't find a place to sleep. They opened their apartments, their houses, their schools, and kindergartens to all families like ours. This is the power of the community. It's like this Bible illustration when the Red Sea is giving you the way to go through to escape from Russia attacks in our case.

JB: Here you are living in uncertainty and fear but to have that community embrace you; this must have been so emotional.

OE: Two weeks ago, we were invited to share our practical experience with resiliency in Oxford, at the family-based conference symposium; it was very unexpected. We visited the symposium online and had an hour to present what we are doing in Ukraine. In the end, we were invited to the award ceremony. EdCamp got a special award for the work we are doing in resiliency. I was so surprised. Dr. Brian Gerrard, the symposium founder, shared why we got this award. Traditionally, resiliency, emotional regulation, body literacy, and attention training—all these soft skills and competencies in schools, abroad in developed countries, taught through special counselors, school psychologists, and coaches, but not by teachers. And we are equipping every teacher in our community with the needed skills and how to teach them to kids and youth. This was the reason behind getting the award. After this, I thought it over and I understood, "Oh, yes! This is really something innovative." We can become the first educational system where teachers, the majority of them, are prepared. They can support themselves, students, and parents and be the trendsetters of these highly needed life skills.

JB: What I am hearing is you look after the teachers, and you respect the teachers. You are giving them the knowledge and skills to collaborate peer-to-peer because it is so powerful to share what they're going through. From a positive psychology perspective that's such a boost, to not feel alone, to be able to share what you're going through. To share the strategies that work and that don't. I wanted to ask you, have a lot of teachers left?

OE: I know some data about educators who left the country, maybe for another profession, temporarily living abroad. It's about twenty-four thousand teachers. I know the data about teachers who have to stay in the occupied territories. They are going through a very hard and challenging experience because of the Russian terror. When occupants enter territories of Ukraine, among the first places they go to are schools. [They] take away and burn books on Ukrainian history, on Ukrainian language, and they force educators to go for professional development activities in their traditional educational system. *(We have a lot of stories from this in our interview series "My war: The lessons for Ukraine and Humanity" mentioned earlier.)* Around eleven thousand teachers stay in the occupied territories, and we know a lot of brave cases of how educators refuse to collaborate and try to escape.

JB: How do you stay mentally strong at a time that there's so much uncertainty? I mean, you have children, and you're not going to wear all of your emotions on your face. I'm a parent too. I understand.

OE: It's a very good question. I am frequently asked what the secret of Ukrainian resiliency is. How are we overcoming all these challenges? Another lesson about the war for myself and for many people around me is that the war reveals what is valuable and what is not. For instance, I am not sure whether I will be able to come back to our family house in Kharkiv. All the belongings, everything we had, remained there. All the materialistic values are secondary, and [there is] this kind of re-evaluation of what is essential and what is not. This is also one of the war lessons: "Your home is where you are. And any part of Ukraine is my home."

Many families are now divided because women and children are going abroad to stay in a safer place and men stay in the country due to the martial law, and a lot of them serve in the army. You see my background on Zoom with a white crow as we are uniting trendsetters and change-makers in Ukrainian education. It is difficult for them to be in their traditional communities, experiment, and find support. EdCamp is like a place of strength, a circle of support with reciprocity that works.

Today's an important day in my professional story. I have a Ph.D. in technical sciences. I taught software engineering students and was keen on mathematics and technology. This was my profession, and I saw myself in this field, but my last ten years have been very bound with education. And I submitted my documents for a post-doctoral program in education. I will be conducting research about the Social, Emotional, and Ethical Learning program and soft skills development. This is like a new chapter of my life. This scientific life within education. Frankly speaking, without the war, I would not have gone in this direction. The war influenced me a lot. Don't wait for a better time to make your dreams the goal. There is a difference between a dream and when you form the aim with the plan to achieve it. There is never a good moment, so I decided to apply this year, and in September, I will be a doctoral student.

JB: I want to ask you about mental health in your country. Here in the United States before COVID, we were already in a mental health crisis. Now with COVID, because of so many factors, we're in a mental health pandemic. You, on the other hand, are experiencing the unimaginable for us. You're in a war, but at some point, was mental health a big issue for students or for adults or was it in the news? Was it talked about?

OE: Of course. Ukraine is not an exception here. We had two hard years of the COVID-19 pandemic, and it influenced all spheres of our lives. This switch to online education was very challenging, and what happened to people whose everyday routine was broken and people got isolated, so we felt the same things as I think any other citizens of the world. But you know what, without this previous COVID-19 experience, it would have been much harder to survive the war because today, we don't have a problem organizing online or blended learning. We are all equipped and prepared. There is a joke in Ukraine: "I wish the COVID times come back" because struggling with the virus is less stressful than the war, although it is still a considerable challenge.

Currently, of course, you will not find a Ukrainian who is not under stress, traumatized, or even experienced PTSD. It's a huge challenge. Therefore, I salute the decision of the First Lady of Ukraine, Olena Zelenska, to make mental health programs her priority, supporting Ukrainians and helping people overcome all these challenges. And you know what, from February 24, the first demand and inquiry to us were, "Please, give us a dose of Social, Emotional, and Ethical learning. Our school wants to participate." Before the war, we were advocating the need for soft skills, resiliency, and emotional management. It was a vast communication where there were schools and educators interested. But now, everybody needs this. And this is a great moment to share this precious knowledge and skills to support the nation, and we have this dream of bringing SEE Learning to every Ukrainian school one day. And we've done a lot for that. We made emotional and ethical competency part of the state curriculum and professional standards.

Now we have the updated toolkit with particular attention to war circumstances. The only thing is to continue doing our work every day and bring this cure, I think in a way, to the schools, and through the school system to the families, the whole nation.

JB: Yes. That is exactly how I feel because if the mental health of teachers isn't in check, and the parents and the students, especially the students, where's their future going to be? You're going to experience so much trauma, especially if they don't feel that there are people they can talk to or resources in schools, or they don't know how to process emotions. That's not going to set them up for success. Because I'm always saying this when I speak to students, the most important thing is really not your grades. It's your mental health.

OE: Yes.

JB: That's going to carry you through in life.

OE: And, you know, I agree absolutely with what you're saying. And therefore, I'm an advocate for this—not trauma-informed, but resiliency-informed education. And the difference is that the resiliency-informed approach is about faith in everybody's capacity to overcome any challenges in one's life. We can survive any experience. This is true. The Ukrainian nation demonstrates with its example not only surviving but enhancing how the world approaches values. When we see this feeling of being united with the democracies of the world, this brings a lot of enthusiasm.

One of my favorite authors offers the radical forgiveness approach. Maybe you know him. This is one of the top books of the EdCamp team library—*Radical Forgiveness* by Colin Tipping. His approach is that every challenge, person, situation, or circumstance in your life is here to teach you, and if you look at this from another angle and reframe it, you will understand that there is no need to forgive. There is only one thing to say, "Thank you." And this is not an easy concept. Mainly, it's hard when you are in a situational war.

It's hard to forgive the Russians for what they are doing. Still, at least in this situation, you can take this energy not to destroy yourself from the inside but to find additional inspiration and motivation to continue living.

JB: Meaning.

OE: Meaning.

JB: Anything else you'd like people to know about EdCamp Ukraine, and also where they can find out more and get involved?

OE: With the help of Elaine Miller-Karas, we launched a resiliency space online supporting activities from the very first day of the invasion. Now, we are transforming this idea to the regular Resiliency Toloka gatherings and you, Janeane, will be one of our guests to join these meetings. And maybe my message to everybody who will be listening to your podcast or reading the book, people from your community of like-minded experts, is if you feel you are willing to share some experience and instruments to support Ukrainian educators, please contact me and join the Toloka encounter. Practitioners, educators, and academics are invited to contribute to this space and participate in an exchange with our educators. The website is EdCamp.ua.

Meet Dr. Michael Yassa

Professor of Neurobiology and Behavior, Neurology, and Psychiatry
– University of California Irvine
Director of the Center for the Neurobiology
of Learning and Memory

"The feeling of loss not just in terms of family members, loved ones, jobs opportunities, but also loss of their daily rhythms, their activities, the kinds of things that they took a lot of comfort in, are now completely compromised."

—Dr. Michael Yassa

Dr. Michael Yassa was a guest on my show on KUCI 88.9 FM, and his work has focused on the mental health needs of students prior to March 2020. He has recognized an increased demand for mental health services to meet student needs over the past several years.

I asked Dr. Yassa to begin by sharing his research regarding student mental health on the University of California Irvine campus.

Michael Yassa (MY): We actually studied this topic actively at UCI because some of our projects are really focused on mental health and young adult community. Even prior to the pandemic, it's clear to us that students on a college campus are generally more vulnerable to mental health concerns. For many of them, it's difficult to understand whether this is a natural part of the stressful cascade of academics, extracurriculars, expectations of family, parents, teachers, and peers, or if there's something more serious. Our counseling center, for example, tends to be very, very busy, but they still don't have the bandwidth to take care of every single student that is struggling with a mental health concern. As a result, many students don't feel that they have sufficient resources. Many don't really understand if they've hit the threshold where they really require assistance or if this is something they should be trying to deal with on their own. So, we're sensitive to those issues because when you do studies on mental health and depression, and you're trying to recruit healthy young adults, and they come in and fill out surveys about their depression symptoms, their anxiety symptoms, and all of a sudden, they qualify as patients rather than healthy controls, you start to see there's a problem.

We certainly saw a lot of that before COVID-19, but it got amplified drastically with the pandemic. The kinds of problems that students were already struggling with, and many of them became worse, and then new problems arose that had to do with isolation, the fear and anxiety around the virus itself. Certainly, the feeling of loss not just in terms of family members, loved ones, jobs opportunities, but also loss of their daily rhythms, their activities, the kinds of things that they took a lot of comfort in, are now completely compromised. So that's a really tough experience to go through, and obviously this is not something that was unique to just college students, but I think it was really amplified in the college student population.

Janeane Bernstein (JB): And I think about the students who come from other countries. They're so excited to come to UCI, and all of a sudden, they have to be remote in their room, their apartment, or dorm.

MY: I talk to students who for the first two years of their college experience (this incredible formative experience that everybody's looking forward to) the transition from high school to college and having to spend all of it remotely from home or just locked up in their dorm rooms. It's extraordinary the impact that that can have, and when you're so looking forward to this experience being such a huge mark on your life, and you're hit with a consequence of the pandemic and hear, "Oh, no, you're not going to be on campus. You're not going to be able to make new friends, new peers, and really soak up this new environment." That can have really devastating consequences, but the students are resilient, and the fact is they are able to now come back to campus and be around their peers. Certainly, the level of comfort with doing that safely is much better now that they can recover from it and still salvage some amount of their college experience. But the fact is, they've lost quite a bit of it. So that's unfortunate.

JB: You mentioned, which has come up in other conversations, "We didn't have the bandwidth or the resources." Do you feel that perhaps there could be some new initiatives—peer-to-peer initiatives—to help one another whereas if something is very serious, students go to the counselor? I know there's WISE PAC (Wellness Initiative in Social Ecology) here at UC Irvine and they were on my show. They're doing great work with their different initiatives, but perhaps there are ways to educate students to work through things with their peers but also know there are resources on campus, and it takes the pressure off the counselors.

MY: You know, Janeane, that's a terrific way to think about it. And I'm glad that you had WISE PAC on the program because they're a great example of what can be done. I'd love to see more initiatives like this across the many schools that we have scattered across all of the institutions of higher education. I think peer mentoring and peer counseling and really kind of getting involved at that level is so crucial, but I think it needs to be an all-hands-on-deck approach. It's not just peers. And it's not just the Counseling Center. We can't just say they're the experts. They're going to take care of the students. We have to be very vigilant about detection and referral, the faculty, the staff, student advising, the deans, the leadership, really everyone should be trained and equipped with the tools for early detection. If a student doesn't come to class three weeks in a row, we should be picking up the phone and saying, "Hey, what's going on?"

We should be very, very aware of what our students are going through now. I know that everybody has limited bandwidth, and we have faculty that teach classes to hundreds of students, but maybe engage the TAs (teaching assistants). Maybe engage at a different level where you have sections, and you have other mentors that are intervening. I think it needs to be a whole-campus approach rather than saying, we're going to have just these isolated efforts within a school or within a department to try to help just a small select segment of students. Because we can't just rely on the counseling center to be the be all and end all; it simply will never have enough resources to take care of everyone. If everybody does their part and everyone has the skills to recognize when something is going on, then I think we can alleviate the burden together.

JB: Perhaps it's a new model of mental health and wellness, where it's a layered approach, but this comes down to policy change because the focus has been academics, "Do really well," and now we need to be a detective looking at issues. If I'm a teacher, and I'm feeling burned out as millions do, I probably don't have the bandwidth. However, this approach should be supported by the university and promoted as a necessity. Be a detective if you see something and troubleshoot; it's a training issue too.

MY: Absolutely. I think you're exactly spot on because right now there isn't that kind of training. I mean, there are resources. There's the red folder that is given to the faculty at UCI, for example, which does have some instructions on how to recognize certain things, how to get students help when they are in need, and where to find those resources. But you ask any faculty member if they know where that is or how to retrieve it, and it's a very small subset that actually know. It's not really part of the overall training that everybody goes through. It is not top of mind, even if it was part of the onboarding. It's not recurrent. So, you have to reemphasize and reinforce those messages. But I think we have to align incentives in the right way. Faculty have to be incentivized. This has to be part of our evaluation process.

Think about how way we communicate to students on the first day with a syllabus. You could put a note in the syllabus that talks about "If you're struggling, if you are worried about mental health, if there are concerns, here's a list of resources for you" that automatically bridges to students and communicates to them that this faculty member cares about the mental health of students. They care, and it says in the syllabus, "Hey, if you don't show up, I'm going to call you. I'm going to come after you and say, what's going on? So, expect that." Sometimes you can get them to be a little bit more proactive and say, "Can I set up a time to chat with you? I'm really struggling. I need some resources. I need some help." And that's much better than having to go and do the detective work to figure out who's in trouble or who needs help.

If people are able to reach out without any fear of judgment or fear that somehow this is going to compromise their performance in class, those kinds of things go a long way. Communicating at the outset about how valuable mental health is for this class or for this major or whatever is really important; it makes a big difference in students' lives and in their fields.

JB: Definitely. It also makes me ask what is whole point of college? Is it just an academic experience? Or is it also how to grow and to be independent and handle the pressures, the ups and downs and to learn what you're going to do when stuff happens. How are you going to take care of yourself? That should be a very important message because they can get straight As. They can caffeinate all they want. They can go-go-go and they can push and they can make honor roll. And then they get out of college, and they're nowhere as far with their mental health and their ability to take care of themselves.

MY: Absolutely, and they are likely to get help and resources in some places that may not be the most reliable, right? And people are on social media trying to expose aspects of their lives and get support from others. But we all know that social media is not really a realistic way to be able to talk about these issues. Sometimes there are things on there that are antithetical to what actually might help and give false hopes, false promises—all sorts of treatments and things out there that may not be the most helpful. So, there's a fear that if we don't have the right level of communication that students will be subject to all sorts of miscommunicated kinds of things and a lot of misinformation that could be detrimental rather than helpful.

We are in a position of privileged authority, at a university setting, in that we do have experts in the field in public health, psychiatry, psychology, and neurobiology and all the areas are kind of related to mental health at large, and we can afford to disseminate that knowledge. We certainly do it in research. We certainly do it in the community, but we need to do a lot more of it for our students on campus, and imbue our faculty, staff, and everybody who interfaces with students, they need the skills and tools to recognize, and at least refer people to the right resources, when they feel that there's a need.

Before you move on to the next chapter, I want to emphasize the critical roles teachers have in our educational systems and their tireless efforts in shaping future generations. Their dedication, training, and expertise should be valued, respected and recognized. Think back to a teacher that made an impact in your own life and why. People who become teachers are passionate about what they do, and some are often discouraged from becoming a teacher. They are certainly not compensated like major league athletes and treated like rock stars, but truthfully, they should be.

What the U.S really needs is a national mental health curriculum that teachers and administrators have as a blueprint in their schools. Ongoing evaluations should be conducted to determine its effectiveness and whether teachers and students are experiencing positive outcomes. Educational settings must promote empathy, compassion, communication, and reduce the exodus of teachers from a profession that has been hard hit. There must also be enough mental health and wellness staff, who are properly trained to listen and address the mental health crisis with actionable steps.

Here are some suggestions for school administrators, counselors, human resources staff, and anyone working in educational settings:

- Assess the mental health and well-being of teachers and create initiatives to nurture their mental fitness and retain them in their essential roles.
- Implement peer support groups, project-based initiatives, preventive mental health programming and resources that represent diverse needs, cultures, races, ethnicities, and marginalized communities.
- Provide mental health education and training using scenario-based learning opportunities so people of all ages know what

to do when they see someone struggling or a situation that might put others at risks (e.g., violent posts on social media, gun related, etc.).

- Get to know your teachers and staff. How are they, *really*? Support their mental health and well-being because they are the glue that holds everything together. Show them you value them and take time to connect and listen.
- Find out their interests, passions outside of school/work. Be fully present and engaged with their willingness to share.
- Encourage students and staff to be open about mental health struggles. Students, especially, want to hear adults share their stories not in a lecture! Share your backstory, something you struggled with, what you do to overcome and move forward.
- Be kind. Be a good listener. Be present. Stop looking at your phone.
- See someone struggling in silence? Reach out. Listen. Provide help. Apathy is not an option.
- Foster open communication about mental health and eliminate stigma.

In the next chapter, you will hear insights and inspiration from the following mental health professionals and advocates:

- *Kelly Davis*—Director of Peer Advocacy, Supports, and Services at Mental Health America
- *Alain Datcher*—Former Executive Director of the Los Angeles County Youth Commission
- *Mallory Gothelf*—Owner/Founder of Find Your/self Boxes
- *Dr. Mitch Prinstein*—Chief Science Officer, American Psychological Association, Distinguished Professor at UNC, Author of *POPULAR*
- *Dr. Raeleen Manjak*—DM/OL, ΔMΔ, CPHR, Director of Human Resources

- *Dr. Bryan E. Robinson*—Psychotherapist in private practice in North Carolina, licensed Marriage and Family Therapist, licensed Clinical Mental Health Counselor, Co-founder and Chief Architect of ComfortZones Digital
- *Kelechi Ubozoh*—a Nigerian-American mental health consultant, advocate, writer, and published author
- *Dido Balla*—Head of Education, MindUP™ | The Goldie Hawn Foundation

CHAPTER 6

Mental Health Professionals and Advocates

*"I really think a champion is defined not by their wins,
but by how they can recover when they fall."*
—*Serena Williams*

Teachers, nurses, and mental health professionals have some of the most crucial roles impacting society. While some weathered the storm, the pressure of the pandemic was physically and emotionally debilitating, and many took to social media to share experiences most of us cannot even fathom. There was no "how to prepare for a pandemic workshop" for teachers, school counselors, and frontline workers. There was a fairly quick announcement that students and staff would be working remotely; there was no prep or planning to prepare them beforehand.

Rates of depression and anxiety escalated for all ages, and healthcare professionals were tapped out from the overwhelming demands for psychologists and psychiatrists. Students and adults who needed to speak to a mental health professional were not seen for a variety of reasons, stemming from socioeconomic and lack of service coverage to lack of trained counselors and therapists. The wait was incredibly long just to get a remote appointment, and unmet needs became the norm. Along with teachers, mental health professionals left their careers as well, and the mental health needs of teens and young adults soared.

We were already living in a mental health crisis pre-pandemic. The term "mental health" represented a stigma not commonly found in a conversation at school or work. Depending on what generation you fit into, your age group might not speak up when facing a personal crisis. You could just "suck it up" and go to work, give an excuse that you need a "sick day," or merely keep your personal struggles to yourself. On the flipside, Generation Z set a precedent in taking a mental health day. It was something they needed to do; they were quite open and honest in prioritizing their health and sharing their struggles on social media.

In March 2020, home lives began to change dramatically. Students had to move back home from college. Parents' stress levels increased because of the economic calamity. Relationships imploded, and work and home life melded under one roof. It was not pleasant at times, and TikTok and Instagram became an entertaining way for people to share their fun and creative sides, including dancing, bread making, and intergenerational games. I found myself very thankful for the technology that brought us connection in a very disconnected and isolating time. I don't know how anyone gets any work done nowadays with the lure of social media.

Grandparents were kept "safe" at a distance and gatherings were all on Zoom. People got creative with their remote time together and how they spent their time during the day. For sure, the pandemic negatively impacted millions of people worldwide, but on the upside, it brought family members together to play games, make homemade sourdough bread, use their shiny new air fryer, learn new hobbies, start exercise routines, and do things that were either new or neglected around the house.

Meet Kelly Davis

Director of Peer Advocacy, Supports, and
Services at Mental Health America

"Teachers have faced really significant barriers over the past couple of years.

That's part of why I think mental health is part of a broader movement for social change and justice and equity."

—Kelly Davis

Kelly Davis is the Director of Peer Advocacy, Supports, and Services at Mental Health America (MHA). She currently works in peer advocacy support and services, where she's involved in promoting peer support, peer certification, youth and young adult leadership, and college mental health.

I reached out to Kelly after keeping up with her thought-provoking posts on LinkedIn. We began the following conversation by her sharing her backstory, how she became a mental health advocate, and her work at MHA. Kelly is doing outstanding work, and she shares a powerful story of her own.

Kelly Davis (KD): I think that the most important part of myself that I bring to my work is my lived experience. Long and short of it, I struggled with my mental health early on. I had my first suicide attempt when I was ten. I spent a lot of my teenage and young adult years in all sorts of treatment. When I was nineteen, I was diagnosed with bipolar disorder and given a really bleak message for what was meant to be the rest of my life.

Janeane Bernstein (JB): Wow!

KD: I was like, okay, yeah, I hear it all the time. All the labels kind of mean different things to different people, but sometimes they can be used in a way that's really disempowering. And that was definitely my experience. So, what happened for me was, I was like, okay, I don't like the path that's been given to me. I'm going to try whatever I can [to change things]. And through that, I got connected to the peer support and recovery movement where I learned that people with my experience were some of the best people that I would ever know and meet. [I learned] other things that I could do to support myself in more empowering ways, like yoga, positive psychology, all of that stuff. I also got access to disability accommodations and was like, wow, everyone should have this. So, that was the journey. Then I went to American University for undergrad, did campus organizing, and interned at the Bazelon Center for Mental Health Law, where I decided I did not want to become an attorney.

And then I started at Mental Health America, and I've been there for the past seven years. I work a lot with youth and young adult activists. I think that's really, really important because there are so many things to learn. And I feel like there's so much pressure, especially when you're younger and just starting in advocacy, to know everything, but no one ever knows everything. The other piece too, is something that I see a lot where people come into mental health advocacy, and they often have a very specific idea of what that means. So, you can only be a mental health advocate if you're a lawyer or a policymaker or a therapist or you know, different types of things. [If you have] a background in journalism, in art—there are so many things that interchange with this work that are really important. I think it's really important to know that we need all types of people to make change.

JB: I remember reading a fantastic article that you had written in the *San Diego Tribune*. And you featured two students, one whom I know is Sriya Chilla. Could you talk a little bit about that article?

KD: Yes, the article was part of the launch of the paper that I also co-authored with Sriya Chilla and Nghia Do, now two freshmen in California. We focused on peer support—how can we empower and work with young people from the most formal to informal levels, certified peer specialist, inpatient mental health, and just talking to your neighbor. [We also discussed] how we can use relationships and the wisdom of young people to address mental health. That is kind of the core idea with the paper. Once I started talking about it, I heard the same thing from lots of other people. Nobody ever asked me what was important to me or what I wanted or what I would do better.

When I would try to advocate for things like peer support programs or say one hour a week in a room is helpful, it wasn't taken seriously. So young people who are living this or people with lived experience of whatever issue know what it's like to go through things. It's really a call to say, you need to listen to the people who you say you're serving, the people who you want to help, because they see stuff that is impossible for you to see. I think that argument was clear pre-COVID. But to say that you understand what it's like to be a high school student during the pandemic....

JB: No way.

KD: Yes, no way. The wildest thing is that one of the things I've always said is mental health is the only product where the consumer is wrong. For some reason, you have to convince people to use something that doesn't make sense for them.

And there's certainly people who push back. I didn't think that I needed an iPhone or Instagram or whatever before I knew what they were, but those were still designed with end users in mind and adapted to their feedback. I think it's changing, but it's really an absurd thing for me. This premise that people with mental health challenges have no idea what would help them is really rooted in a lot of outdated ways of thinking, and then when you intersect with different forms of marginalization, including being a young person, it's worse.

JB: Besides peer-to-peer initiatives, what else do you think we can do to become better humans? Meaning, you know, become more compassionate, more in tune, more open and accepting?

KD: Yeah, that's an interesting question. This past year, we have a Youth Mental Health Leadership program at MHA. I'm working with members to write a paper, and it's kind of this idea of power. So, it's like power within, power with other people, and power to do something. I think there's really important dynamics when you look at somebody who thinks more like on a societal or like community level. There are community norms, there are policies that impact how people are or are not supported and their mental health and have really punitive requirements for college students who, for whatever reason, have to miss a deadline or miss a class. There are policies there. And then there's also making sure that people have access to lots of different pathways to wellness, right?

So yes, you can have someone to talk to. Do you have something using technology that's supportive and teaching you skills that you can use yourself? Do you understand or learn about journaling or art? Do you have access to different communities who care about the same things as you that can be therapeutic, whether that's sports, social justice, the gym, or yoga? You know, there's so much more.

I think one of the shortcomings of how we frame mental health as a "this is a therapy thing" discounts most of people's lives and what's important to them. So, I think it's really a dynamic and people should have access to all of these different things that help them feel more whole, not just, you know, being able to talk to someone. It is helpful, but if you can't change the policies that are negatively impacting your life, and if you can't do the things that make you feel good and help you grow, that's missing the whole thing. It is not just about peer; it's about creating healthy people and conditions where people can thrive and be healthy.

Kelly shared some learning moments taught by the experience of living in a pandemic. I have heard others share similar thoughts, but I loved how she framed her insights.

KD: I feel like in talking about learnings from COVID, there's a lot of things that we're unlearning in mental health, one of which being psychology's deep need to be a hard science. Actually, a lot of the things that help and are therapeutic are not just kind of traditional talk therapy; [there is] this idea that art is not important. These things aren't important. What did everyone do to escape during COVID, right?

JB: Yes.

KD: Engage in art. Engage in reading and film and all these things. I think it's really exciting to see that, and listening to people means that we're going to take more seriously the way that we've always done things does not really meet people's needs.

JB: Yes, I fully agree. And I remember people saying, oh, I just want to go back to normal. And I'd say, normal is not healthy.

Kelly: Right. I will say, though, it's really important for people who care about health advocacy to double down because I'm seeing a lot of, "We thought everything was going to change for mental health" stuff, kind of go back to pre-COVID.

JB: Give me an example.

KD: I feel like people were, "Oh, it's okay to take care of yourself; it's okay to share the hard things that are going on in your house. It's okay to have people running around in the background of your Zoom." And I feel like it's all kind of shifting back again. I've even seen that in work with college students. One of the things that's been really hard in the disability community is a lot of accommodations, like flexibility with attending classes, being able to attend virtually class recordings, that students have been denied pre-COVID were available for everyone during COVID and then went away.

JB: (gasp) What?!

KD: Yes. It depends on your accommodations. Professors have a lot of leeway in what they allow in their classes, but I think it's really important to not lean back. It's an ongoing process and maybe a fight that resonates with me as an activist, but you really need to continue to engage and continue to push. I've been thinking about this a lot and hearing a lot. In some ways it feels like everybody just completely decided that we aren't going to talk about the past couple of years, which I get is the trauma response.

But one of the things that a lot of clinicians and researchers were saying before the pandemic was that people really come together during a crisis, during a natural disaster. And then you see once you get like six months afterward, people kind of start falling apart. And I think we talked about mental health during the pandemic. There were really bad issues, but the resources weren't there for unpacking what we just all hopefully are mostly done, but what we've all lived through.

JB: Yes. I couldn't agree more. Because first in schools, there weren't enough resources to help students. There weren't enough counselors. There wasn't really a strong heads up, like "Let's prep for a pandemic." And then I heard students going back to school and they had lost a grandparent, a parent. There's been so many articles, I'm sure you've seen how many kids have lost parents and how traumatic that is.

I'm impressed with Mental Health America. Every day there's a post about mental health and something very specific that people should pay attention to, and today's article was, which is not a shocker, that students aren't doing well academically.

KD: There are a few things. One is—we don't have collective spaces for grief. One is school, even pre-COVID. And also, it's an equity issue, right? Where you are and where you live and what your racial or ethnic or class background impacts you. But from what I hear on the one end of things with the pandemic, furthering that high school is like a professional prep track, where the competitiveness of getting into college is so absurd right now. Fourteen-year-olds are having to think about things like they're like twenty-two.

It's just ridiculous. The pressure on young people is absurd; it doesn't make sense to me how all these like looking at these schools, every school's entrance seems like you have to have like a 4.2 GPA.

JB: Come on!

KD: It's absurd. Yeah, I think that's what is happening. I think that that ties into economics and all these broader social issues. But I also think too, one of the things that's really challenging right now is that we're about to launch a program working with current and recent high school students to advocate for mental health policy for K–12. And it's hard because you have this knowing and sometimes some folks [have] lived experience of how hard it is. And a lot of schools can't hire teachers.

Teachers have faced really significant barriers over the past couple of years. That's part of why I think mental health is part of a broader movement for social change and justice and equity. It's kind of absurd to only think about well, you need to add these mental health things in here. Teachers are so overwhelmed, so underpaid, so kind of traumatized from the past couple of years that they're like, we can't even fill our roles for teachers. How are we going to do all this extra stuff? It's all interconnected. Mental Health Advocacy, I think, is important too. If you're doing mental health advocacy, it's important to learn about and understand how that intersects with all different parts of advocacy.

JB: Yes, it's interesting talking about teachers because I was reading that over three hundred thousand teachers have left the profession since 2020. That's a massive number.

KD: So how do we address childhood mental health when our schools are so toxic or non-supportive that you can't find teachers?

JB: And I look at the reasons why they're leaving. They're not respected by the administration, the parents; they are not compensated enough. There are issues of what they can and cannot teach. There's so much....

KD: Yeah. And it points to a cultural under-emphasis in, like caring for other people, and how that's valued because it's the same thing with the mental health professional workforce where it's like, we need more therapists. We need more of this. And it's obscene. The amount of debt relative to the workload and the rates that therapists are reimbursed by insurers. So, we have a kind of caring professions who are not cared for, and it's a really hard balance as an advocate because you have to advocate for these changes. But at the same time, there's all of these structural and historic barriers that have created what we're seeing right now.

JB: Yes. So, as you said, we have therapists who have left the profession, so we have greater demand for therapists. We don't have enough people to help the people who need it.

KD: Yeah, and I think, you know, tech and peer-to-peer approaches are certainly important parts of how we address and improve mental health and create more mentally healthy communities. I think it also doesn't make sense that our framework to the public is you either have good mental health or you have to go see a therapist or a psychiatrist. There's way more complexity in between those two ideas.

Investing in the workforce, I think, is really important. And it's not the only thing.

JB: Right. And I think it does come back to being better humans. In a sense, because I don't think we've been thoughtful enough to one another. I think, you know, at times, we live a very individualistic way of living and if we could just maybe put ourselves in other people's shoes, whether it's that teacher or that doctor or nurse or whomever, right. So many people have been hit so hard by the pandemic.

KD: Yeah, that is what is the saying. It's simple, but it's not easy. Like so many people, one of the most powerful experiences, or one of the most, I guess, perspective-changing experiences that I've had in my mental health advocacy is I helped create a youth empowerment training and one of the pilots they did was in South Dakota. Some young people who were in the juvenile justice system participated and were bused in. One of the participants cried and said, "No one has ever asked me what matters to me before."

JB: (gasp) Oh!

KD: Especially when you're talking about young people, like what matters to you, knowing your name. I can't remember where else I read it. Some young people go days without—I could cry—someone saying their name. The structural change and policy and financing—they're all important, but there are so many basic human things that we can do. I also think systems need to be a lot better at it too.

JB: I agree.

KD: Like individual people's lives.

JB: Yes. So, you think it's a policy change, a system change…

KD: It has to be all of it. Unfortunately, the world is really complicated, and I think it's important as people in a movement to really understand and value that we need all different types of change because sometimes it can be like "You're so far removed. You don't understand what needs to happen on the ground. You know, you don't understand that your demands are unreasonable because all this stuff," and I think we need more spaces for people to feel like they have an entry point to learn about things and define where they fit in because we don't need more divisiveness. We need as many people as possible to care about this and take action. I think with COVID, there's no one who is not touched by this.

JB: I agree completely. I have focused a lot lately on how Gen Z is doing. They're saying, "If they don't deal with their mental health now, where are they going to be as adults?"

KD: And we don't know the impact—we have no data to compare what living through a pandemic does long term. I think people understand how different the world is from when a lot of the research and frameworks that we have and used were first developed in individual one-on-one therapy in an office. The world is just different now.

JB: Completely. I think more people, again, need to be more empathetic and compassionate and step outside of their own lives if they're able to, if they haven't felt like they've really struggled very much. I've heard people say, "Well, now that the pandemic is in our rearview mirror...."

KD: (Laughter)

JB: Kelly, I can't believe it when people say "Well, now that the pandemics behind us..." and I would disagree.

KD: And everybody's had that experience, and it just reminds me of the research that stigma reduction campaigns can be effective, but the best way to reduce stigma is to be in proximity to someone who talks about their mental health. There was a survey that came out from the Healthy Minds Network that said that for the overwhelming majority of young people, what would help them feel more comfortable talking about their mental health was not having celebrities but having people in their lives talk about it. I think it's undersold how much identifying and sharing your story, and all those things, can have on the world around you, too.

Meet Alain Datcher

Former Executive Director, Los Angeles
County Youth Commission

"We have to call this current culture on the carpet and identify what the pandemic and all of its tertiary effects are. What opportunity has that now allowed us as policymakers, as advocates, and members of the media, to unpack, to unlearn about our young people, and then how do we respond?"

—Alain Datcher

Several months ago, I received an email regarding an online event led by Alain Datcher, who at time was the executive director of the Los Angeles County Youth Commission. The Commission focuses on youth-centered initiatives created and led by the ideas of youth and young adults.

I met Alain after attending my first Los Angeles County Youth Commission webinar, and this is the same event where I heard Rocket Garcia share her traumatic story. Alain began by describing his role as the Los Angeles County Youth Commissioner.

Alain Datcher (AD): I would say sometimes I have the best job in the world. I oversee one of the very first government advisory bodies led by and centered on youth and young adults. Essentially what we do is represent the voices of Los Angeles County's over two million youth and advise our Board of Supervisors, department leaders, agency leaders, and community-based organizations on the issues or the recommendations and ideas that young people have; this can include anything related to transportation, mental health, public health, and education. I help oversee and build a strategy so that we can get things done and achieve goals on behalf of our young people.

Janeane Bernstein (JB): I first heard about you and your organization when I joined one of your webinars a few months ago. I was so impressed with the youth that you had joining you. One thing that struck me was when some of the adults were saying, "We're not listening. We're not kind. We're not compassionate." What I love about what you're saying is you're *actually* listening to these youth. What do they need? What do they want? In that process, we can become better humans and move out of this mental health pandemic or have a better understanding of how to move forward in a positive direction.

Alain: You know, Janeane, I'm not sure who coined the term radical listening. But that is really what we try to practice. As a leader, I've tried to instill a culture that is obsessed with communication. We are obsessed with trying to engage our young people. We are obsessed with trying to figure out what they are saying and how they are saying it. Where are the spaces that our young people are sharing their voices? And essentially what we're saying is providing a mirror back to the government into these decision-makers, into these mental health providers, into all of these communities who care about young people. We are here to say, guess what? Where are you engaging the young people in your midst now? Tell us what they are saying.

Far too often, a lot of these departments don't know how to affect these young people, even though they have millions of dollars' worth of programs and services. Even though we have dozens of staff, such as psychiatric social workers, staff from the Department of Mental Health or the Department of Public Health, social workers in the Department of Children and Family Services, we all need to be trained in engaging ways on "how do I effectively communicate in order to serve them more effectively."

On that panel, you heard it right. People said, "I just wish you would listen, not necessarily for agreement, but understanding." Yes, we would. Listen to me in here and believe me when I say I need this or believe me when I say that I'm struggling; this is the underside of what we don't ever really talk about. These kids that are in foster care or are currently behind bars, which is also who we are going out and talking to—it is devastating to see the ways in which these young people are just marginalized, left out of sight, out of the public discourse around some of the issues facing young people, especially in the mental health field.

JB: Definitely. You and I had talked another time. Imagine if someone asked one of these youth, "So, why did you steal?" And you start uncovering all these reasons: "My mom is a single mom, she lost her job, we don't have enough food," and so on. There are so many issues right now with mental health.

AD: Yes. When we talked about that analogy it just sparked so many other things. That is currently what we are dealing with here in Los Angeles. There is a spike in crimes, especially petty theft, and in felony theft. One of our youth commissioners was live on our local FOX News station and spoke about all of these conversations that are happening right here. There are lawyers that are part of the conversation of the District Attorney, and there's all of these different groups. No young people are at the table saying, "This is what we think is happening."

We've just spent two and a half years of disruption in significant loss, and we have not collectively mourned. We have not collectively addressed; we have not collectively strategized. We have not collectively, I would say, built the public awareness around what have we just gone through. What the heck are we still in? How do we know we're going to be on the other side of this? Economically? Is it going to be communally?

Because I can tell you what our young people are saying. There was an eighth grader we were talking with during one of our mental health listening sessions. This eighth grader said, "When the pandemic started up, [I was] just about to go into middle school as a fifth grader. I didn't even have a normal graduation. By the time I'm fully back into school where we're not having any disruptions, I'm an eighth grader." So, she has missed her entire middle school development experiences. I imagine back to when we were in middle school, all the things that you needed to know, like building friendships, maybe taking a tough class, engaging with a tough teacher. All of these positive developmental milestones that are just myths are just disrupted or non-existent.

JB: There's so much depression, anxiety, suicides, suicidal thoughts. I feel that policymakers are missing an opportunity by not talking to today's youth to really understand what the needs are. I mean, it really sounds like marketing. You want to find out what the customer needs, go to the customer. Listen. Do focus groups as you were saying.

AD: Yes, and that is the bare minimum. Let's just be honest. Bare minimum is when we listen, and then we will be able to react or respond in substantial ways. We use the analogy for business. There is no successful business that does not engage or listen to their customers. We just need to just do some old-fashioned marketing research. More specifically, we have to call this current culture on the carpet and identify what the pandemic and all of its tertiary effects are. What opportunity has that now allowed us as policymakers, as advocates, and members of the media, to unpack, to unlearn about our young people, and then how do we respond? Those are the types of conversations we need to have and those are the types of conversations I want to be focused on. That is where I think you'll find solution-eering with our young people. That's what energizes our young people around mental health.

I am so surprised day in and day out by just how energetic our young people are when we're talking to them about tough situations like mental health, like saying how could we help support you and your mental health journey? What worked, what doesn't? You'll hear not just listening, but you also hear why talk therapy is the only thing we have. These are these are young people that are creative and want to do arts and animal therapy, drumming. They want therapies that are that are culturally and gender informed for them so that they can actually be more responsive, that wealth of service providers is preventative, that helps keep our young people potentially out of other harmful diagnoses like depression, anxiety, and potential suicidal ideation. That is a preventative measure when we say, "We heard you."

Talk therapy isn't the only thing we should be offering, so let's go and find those services. Let's not define who should provide those services all the time. It may not be a licensed clinical social worker, but this could be a pastor in a local Black or Brown community that's well-respected and well-regarded. [It could be] a coach, a dance instructor, a yoga instructor. And then how do we use public funding in order to fund those types of services? The young people want those and are engaged in those.

That is where I really want us to truly reimagine what our services can be. And to put a full court press on, let's get those services out there. Let's identify and let's market those things. And then we also got to talk about the cultural stigma, right? Because we can provide all the services we can provide. We can get those services; we can market them effectively. But then let's talk about what happens at that home. The young person might want those services, the mom or dad may have stigmas around, right? Education. We got to talk about a two, three, four generational approach around mental health and why it's so important. What are the other factors of why mental health are so important? I can tell you I can't afford a therapist if I'm struggling to pay rent. That is happening right? This moment. So, we do talk about mental health. We have to talk about it in a much larger context around just caring for our most vulnerable.

Essentially, that is what we're doing, and our young people are at the center of that. In any major social determinants of health, when we actually center our young people around it, you hit education, mental health, public health, and communal factors. It just really drives the ripple effect across our communities. And we can say, "Where are young people going to be in 2025 and 2026?" That's where our solutions need to be geared toward right now.

These are the kids that will be in college soon. How are universities prepared to engage these young folks now and where they will be in five or so years? One of the factors that I think you continue to highlight is the well-being of a young person, but we also have to talk about who isn't mentioned in these discussions, right? Our parents. Our caretakers. How are we supporting them? Even more, how are we supporting the teachers?

We know at least in LA County, 80 percent of our young people get their mental health services as it's tied to their educational or community-based organizations, so these kids are getting their mental health through a school counselor or through a school therapist, or potentially again, through a coach and what not. This is where their well-being is centered. What strategies do we have to support these folks, as we know, now schools have kind of taken on a different and a dual role.

So not only do I need to care about class instruction and make sure I'm meeting these metrics, I have kids who, again, have an increased amount of anxiety or depression, kids who are now exhibiting behavioral factors. How do we do that without expelling our young people without further marginalizing, or penalizing our young people who are suffering in the midst of this unspeakable, unspeakable, unknowable pandemic?

No one thought this was going to be this difficult. I remember getting an email saying we'll be back in a couple of weeks, you know, and a couple of weeks turned into a couple of months and then years. That is the story of so many different people. Yes, for young people in the families that they live in the communities that they reside in, and the folks that they care about, we have to talk about that ecosystem. How do we strengthen that? And again, in the federal to the state and local government, what is the role that we must play in mental health as a part of a larger piece?

You talked about the curriculum too, Janeane, and I think, just as we have physical education, we have to talk about mental education. I mentioned our listening sessions. In one of our listening sessions with some youth from Burbank, they talked about a best practice. They have non-instruction days, but the day will be focused on well-being and mental health. So instead of having in-class instruction, they actually have teachers and outside organizations come in just to talk about well-being in the screen.

You're still learning, it's still in a community, but it's one that is now centering and valuing the importance of your mental health and your well-being as a part of your larger learning. To me, that shouldn't be innovative. If you talk about where young people are, you'll shift your curriculum. Our young people are telling us in so many different ways, "We are hurting. We are not okay. Things are not normal." So why should our approaches still be the one that we were using pre-pandemic? We cannot use pre-pandemic solutions for post-pandemic realities. It just won't work. We have to rethink, reimagine, call to carpet, and take into account these current structures that just aren't working for us.

JB: Yes. One thing that I keep in mind, because I do a talk about the science of happiness and resilience, is to engage, interact, and listen with whomever I'm talking to. Because I feel that we need preventative education. And by that, I mean, as you said, look at the impact on the teachers who are, by the way, leaving the profession, and counselors. No one was prepared for this. If you provide preventative measures, peer-to-peer opportunities for students to work with one another as well as go to a counselor, it's a win-win in the long term.

AD: Yes, it is. Counselors are already having these conversations. I have a friend, and she's a school counselor. And she talked years ago about the struggles and the differences that she was seeing in our young people before the pandemic. So, these trends were already going up. There were stresses around grades, colleges, and social media. Then you factor in other situations. In our African American communities, for example, there was already a high rise of anxiety, depression, and also suicides among Black teens. We weren't talking about these things, but our counselors on the frontlines were seeing this. As administrators and as policymakers, where are our ears right now?

If the experts are telling us what they need, telling us where the issues are, what is the issue? What must we unpack in order for us to be able to provide solutions, provide those resources? To me, it's a question of will; it really is. What is our political will in order to get these things done and achieved on behalf of our young people? What's practical, and what's idealistic?

Now, will we have robust mental health curriculum in LAUSD (Los Angeles Unified School District), one of the largest school districts? Probably not overnight, but I do think that we can start to support local schools. We have,

I believe, eighty school districts in our county. I'm sure we can start to encourage more school districts and build tools and build a network of sharing, right? Those are the types of practical solutions we can be now in order to say this is what Burbank is doing. This is what this local, smaller school district is doing in order to help the young people, and then again, practice radical listening. Halting sometimes in class instruction in order to just have spaces in places for young people to share their thoughts or ideas.

That in and of itself is a part of healing. Because one thing is we're more accountable with knowledge. With knowledge comes accountability, so I can't continue to ignore a situation that I know about, unless I'm really now saying, "Well, this just isn't that important to us." And our young people are seeing that, and they're still sharing their ideas and their thoughts. They're just not doing it in places and spaces now that they don't feel are listening. They're not sharing sometimes their concerns or their thoughts or their frustrations at home because parents aren't listening. Being honest, right? They're not sharing them in schools because some of their teachers or administrators aren't listening. So, we have to really talk about that as well.

And I also think that when we practice that radical listening, what comes about that is what then will we do with these ideas and phenomenal solutions that young people are sharing? What is this pile of great ideas and deep-seated needs? What do we do with those needs, other than have to build stronger partnerships? Have to engage the media. Talk about this! This should be front and center.

Why isn't our media talking about this? We talk about the reactions, but we don't necessarily talk about the rising crime, we don't talk about the rise of suicidal ideations that can be tied to. I'll get off my soapbox, but these are the types of things that we've got to lean on our community partners, as well. Everyone has a voice in this, and everyone has a place at the table. I think you opened up with a larger context around the role of a mandated reporter. I know in LA County, my colleague, Dr. Tamara Hunter, the executive director of the Commission for Children and Families here in LA County. One of all the things that she has been highly talking about is not only the use of data and information to drive our decisions, but even more so shifting from a mandated reporter where it is just really kind of investigative to mandated *supporter* where you are trained to provide, like, "Hey, if I see something now here is the wealth of support I already know about because I've been trained, not just to report the need, and then kind of make sure that I've met my obligation, right?" How do we actually create conditions where a young person you're concerned about will get the support that they need? That is the shift of thinking that we are trying to push here in LA County, and I think we've been able to shift some of the narratives over the last year or so.

JB: You know, I think you talked about students missing milestones, and I think about what that does to their self-esteem, their mental health, their emotional health, and I feel that this, as you said, is an opportunity for immense change and to really listen, pay attention, and figure out how can we take what we're learning in the mental health pandemic and create positive change.

AD: Yes, there's nothing much I can add to that only that, you know, preach it. I think, again, I want to reiterate that the conversations are happening in places and spaces, but we also have to go to where our young people are in our communities are.

You brought up that at certain schools they say, "Well, we have a day devoted to it and we have this." That is not enough. Why? Because the young people will tell you that's not enough. And like you said, it must be baked into, organically woven into how we instruct, how we care, how we discipline, how we hold our young people accountable, the full lifecycle. And then also continue to highlight the young people who aren't here, who we don't see, which are those kids who are in foster care, in residential treatment facilities, or currently incarcerated, who, by the way, are also struggling with the same anxiety, the same amounts of depression.

They're exacerbated when one person is incarcerated; they're exacerbated when a young person is away from their community, from their family. And they're in these home-like settings, but ultimately, they're not home, or they don't feel at home. And so, I think that is also what we must continue to talk about it. It's not just who's speaking but also who's not. Making sure that they get their voice and at some point, in time, get an opportunity to be shared.

I was in a juvenile hall facility here in LA County about a month ago, and I had a chance to sit down with a young man and talk to him. He's currently incarcerated, and he's been there for about seven years. Talked with him, sat down, kind of like how we were face-to-face, getting to know who he was and sharing a little bit about myself. And at the end of that conversation, one of the most powerful things he said was, "Alain, will you come back? And will you write me?" This young man on the outside, you'd be like, "He's arrested.

He's committed these heinous offenses. Throw away the key." But when we got there, we got face-to-face, this was a man who wanted to do better and was in tune with his mental health. He knew about some of the traumas he had faced and the adverse childhood experiences he had faced. And what he wanted was community. What he wanted was a sense of connection. What he wanted was someone who could believe in him. And I think that is at the heart of how we support our young people. It's not radical to say I will support a young person, no matter their circumstances, I'll be here to support them no matter their circumstances. To reiterate that, that's the type of culture that we're building. That's the type of community I'd like to continue to push toward.

Meet Mallory Gothelf

Owner and Founder, Find Your/self Boxes – Boston, MA

"When you're present with that phone away, you're saying I'm giving you my full attention.

That does wonders and feels like someone's listening to me and my voice, my thoughts, my opinions."

—Mallory Gothelf

When my daughter was having a rough time in college, I thought I would send her a care package, but what did that mean, exactly? Was there a company that made care packages for college students that didn't include movie candy and flavored popcorn for temporary joy? Nothing was standing out in the sea of online businesses, until I found *Find Your/self Boxes*, a unique company with a purpose-driven mission—self-care packages for the mind, body, and soul founded by Mallory Gothelf, who has lived experience and a passion to help others. Since then, Mallory has been a guest on my series Outside the Box. I am thrilled to share her backstory with you. Here's how Find Your/self Boxes came to be.

Mallory Gothelf (MG): I was in a workplace that didn't necessarily prioritize mental health care, and at the same time, when a coworker would take off for mental health reasons, there would be a lot of talk in the office behind their back, speculating about this person's work ethic. It made me uncomfortable because I was like, what if I need to take off for that or I leave every Tuesday at four to go to therapy? Are people saying the same things about me when I walked out of this room? There was still some shame and stigma, and I was still afraid to say, "I'm taking off for an adult health day. I would say, I'm not feeling well physically. I always had to let them know that it was something physical because I still felt some shame about being honest. But there are times when my mental health just acts up. I'm not doing well, and that was very much the reality pre-pandemic. A part of me felt like stepping into a different identity when I went into my workplace. I had to be someone who didn't struggle with mental health because I didn't want anyone to look down upon me or judge my work ethic or my ability to be in that room.

Mallory explains the stigma and discomfort society still feels around mental health, and the lack of acceptance and openness is detrimental. She began by sharing how the mental health pandemic came to be.

MG: I think it's a lot of factors. I think one of them is simply that we sweep these things under the rug. We want to talk about it, but the second we say something that steps a little too much, maybe not so lightly, people are like, "Oh, no, that's not the thing." They're free to be judged, and they're afraid of labels being used around them. I think the big ones are "crazy" or "out of control" or whatever you want to label it.

As soon as someone starts to use those labels for people, they're like, "Let's not talk about mental health anymore," because they're afraid of being stigmatized or put in a box. I think our silence continues to perpetuate a lot of the mental health struggles; it doesn't give people the opportunity to go get help. In the same vein, I think when people are ready to get help, help isn't necessarily incredibly accessible. I know for me personally, I was very fortunate that growing up, especially when I was under my parent's insurance, I was afforded opportunities to go into treatment facilities and get the help that I needed, or I could afford the medications at the time that I needed them. And a lot of people don't have that. They don't have the ability to enter facilities, they can't afford medications, so they're stuck on their own trying to figure it out.

Even if we do want to get help, and we are having these conversations, not everyone can access the things that they need to access to get better. And that's on a systemic level of what our healthcare system looks like; that's a much bigger problem as well. Mental healthcare cannot be a priority because people are too afraid to talk about it. And if more people start talking about it, especially people with influence, and we're even just a bunch of people who have influence, it can't drown out our voices. That's when shame starts happening. And it needs to happen. It needed to happen two years ago, and it needs to happen now. It's that saying, "This should have happened yesterday," but it didn't, so now we make it happen today.

Janeane Bernstein (JB): I think about the mental health of Asian Americans, Black people, mental health of BIPOC, LGBTQ—so many people have been impacted.

MG: Oh, absolutely. And those communities especially because on top of just the mental health, navigating through their day to day lives, or it's just more difficult for them, the way that you know, the oppression that they face, the discrimination that they face. It adds another layer of complexity for them when they're trying to heal, and that especially needs to be made a priority. Those communities who are facing such oppression really need to be put in the spotlight and be given access to resources to really help heal.

I asked Mallory to share how she built her business, as a way to help others the way she wanted to be helped.

MG: I really started this business because I know how difficult it can be to want to help someone you love who's struggling but not having the language for it, not knowing what to say. I know that my family, when I was first struggling, would walk on eggshells around me. It wasn't that they didn't love or care about me. They just didn't have the education around mental health to feel comfortable like sitting down and talking to me like a political person. I think when we talk, we are more comfortable talking about certain physical health challenges. We're more open, and we feel like we're able to spend some words with mental health. People feel so afraid that as a gesture they can say I'm here to support you.

These boxes were really made to show up at your door and say, I see you in your struggle. And I love you and when you want to talk and when you are ready to talk, I'm here for you. And I pair that with products that I find really helpful in my day-to-day self-care and which other people also find helpful. The boxes really tried to focus on the five senses, helping people ground themselves in the here and now, and also just adding joy into their day. I think a lot of times we take away that idea that we make healing so serious that we forget that healing can be playful. Healing can be something where you can kind of get in touch with all of your emotions. We try to add products that are kind of fun that evoke that sense of playfulness and childlike kind of [wonder] in life. We wanted to introduce that as a way to embrace that feeling. It's going to be a journey and it's going to be lifelong, but it can be fun, and it can be something that you don't have to dread every single day or something you don't have to spend a ton of money on.

We try to make the boxes really affordable so that people realize self-care isn't just the grand gesture of, you know, going to a spa all day and spending a ton of money. It can be something as simple as sitting down with a tea and just enjoying it, savoring it for that moment or playing with our aromatherapy doh and just sitting in that moment of just playing almost like with Play Doh. So, it's simple things that you can incorporate into your day to day. I'm here in this moment. I'm taking care of myself in a way that feels good. And reminding yourself that healing is possible in those small moments.

JB: It's really amazing because along the journey of helping yourself, you figured out a way to help other people with this wonderful focus on self-care prioritized in your life.

MG: I used to ask, "Why me?" a lot. Why do I have to go through this? Why do I have to struggle? And I think when I started realizing that I could reach back and help other people so they didn't necessarily feel so alone in their struggle, that's when I stopped asking why me? I think it gave purpose to my struggle and my illness and gave it meaning. So I didn't have to ask those questions at night, and I now had a way to look at it and say, "Okay, if I did have to struggle, if I do have to go through these things, I'm going to find a way to use it, you know, to better my community and better society." And that to me feels like even though I wouldn't necessarily wish depression on myself or any other person, it gives it meaning and it makes it feel worthwhile to have gone through. You're really saying, I see you, I feel you. I empathize because I've been down that road.

JB: How do you think we can become better humans right now? As far as in schools and businesses, and the way we live our life?

MG: Yeah, that's a really wonderful question. I think sometimes we just listen to one another and just ask one another, how are you doing today? And really mean that when you ask it and listen to the person's response. I think if we're open to having conversations and get less focused on what's going on, on social media, or in the news, or constantly being plugged in, but taking the time to be present in the company of other people, I think it opens the door for us to have more of these conversations. And we can really be there for other people.

One of my favorite things to do is when a friend tells me they're going through a hard time, I ask, "Do you want feedback, or do you just want me to listen?" I think it opens the door for us to have really meaningful conversations. I'm not doing something that's going to push them away. I'm giving them what they're looking for. Because I think we're quick to give answers and solutions that we think are going to be helpful, and it's kind of closing the door to conversation because people aren't feeling like they're being heard or listened to in that moment. So, that's something that I've employed with my friends when they're like, "Can I talk to you about something?" I'll immediately ask, "Is this a feedback time or is this just me listening?"

They tell me we have these really powerful conversations because I can be there in that moment. I give them exactly what they're looking for. And so, I think if we are willing to sit with one another and be open and be vulnerable, and listen—really listen, we can be better to one another. I know it sounds so simplistic, but it really can be that simple. It's those little things that all kind of snowballed together for greater change.

I even find with friends who are my age, they'll see a text light up while I'm talking, and I see them look over at it. Immediately, [I feel like I] don't want to continue the conversation. I don't because I'm in the middle of expressing something that's difficult for me to express. And I feel like I'm not holding their attention. I noticed I pull back and don't really want to have the conversation anymore. When you're present with that phone away, you're saying, "I'm giving you my full attention." That does wonders and feels like someone's listening to me and my voice, my thoughts, my opinions. You matter to someone, and that can be a real difference maker, especially when you're struggling with something like depression that makes you feel kind of worthless. The soul, the soul gesture, saying like, "I'm going to listen to you and give you my full attention." You're like, okay, maybe I do matter. That is a really, really important thing for someone to know especially when they're struggling.

Meet Dr. Mitch Prinstein

Chief Science Officer, American Psychological Association,
Distinguished Professor at UNC, Author of *Popular*

*"Kids are embedded in systems—a school system, a home system,
a community system. Just figuring out what's going on for kids is
much more complex. Treating kids is treating the climate—the
entire environment or systems in which kids live."*

—Dr. Mitch Prinstein

I first met Dr. Mitch Prinstein as a guest on my show talking about
his book, *Popular*. Most recently, I heard him speaking on a Los
Angeles radio station. When the host asked listeners to call in and
share their views on education and the pandemic, I was able to
speak live with Dr. Prinstein. As you can imagine, I had a lot to say!
Afterward, I invited him to be a guest on Outside the Box and be part
of this book. Here's what he had to say about the effect of technology
on mental health, the mental health pandemic, policy changes, and
moving forward.

Janeane Bernstein (JB): In the pandemic, technology had
its upside obviously. I can't imagine if we weren't able to
connect virtually in meaningful ways. The downside is that
we're missing out, making comparisons, and focusing on
body image, and so on. What are you seeing in your work?

Mitch Prinstein (MP): You're absolutely right. It's so
interesting how we have this new relationship with technology
that was driven by necessity during the pandemic. And we're
seeing some of that parallel in the research literature. So
yes, it turns out that kids who use technology to connect
with friends during the pandemic reported less loneliness.
There was a benefit. Absolutely. There are a lot of ways that

social media or digital technology can be used for good. Finding a number of areas of bad and at this point, it's really preliminary work because it takes a long time to do research and this stuff changes really fast, but social comparisons is a piece of it. Exposure to harsh online content is another big piece that we're seeing for marginalized groups. There's a lot of exposure to discrimination; it's more frequent, and it's harsher than you see in its offline counterpart. There are all these pro-maladaptive behavior sites, pro-anorexia, pro-cutting sites that admonish kids for doing the right thing, really sanction them for talking with their parents, and encourage them, "You have to cut, you have to do it more, show your pictures."

JB: That is sick!

Mitch: It's really scary. As a parent and as a scientist, no matter how I look at it, it freaks me out.

JB: Yes, because it perpetuates this situation that is not healthy.

MP: We should not be making maladaptive behavior cool. "We're going to make you have to log out of our chat. We're going to send you imagery and have a worldwide audience to discourage you from adaptive coping strategies." That's horrible.

JB: With the recent gun violence in Uvalde, Texas, I remember looking at tweets. ABC News had interviewed students, and the students said, "We saw this kid come to school with scratches on his face and we said, 'What happened?' He said, 'Oh, I did it. I liked the way it looked.'" They didn't do anything with that information, and maybe didn't know what to do, and they were frightened. So, my feeling is, Mitch, we need an overhaul of the educational system. Here we adopted STEM and STEAM, but not mental health, into curriculum. To me, mental health is the priority right now, and should have been.

MP: Absolutely. There are so many things that we can teach, and we can teach very quickly, you know, in twenty minutes, half an hour, which could provide a lifetime of prevention benefits. I often think about the time that I was in kindergarten, and someone came in and taught us how to brush our teeth. Every spot that we missed turned red because we had a tablet or something like that, and in twenty minutes, we were given a lifetime prevention exercise to avoid cavities. If you give psychologists twenty minutes to go to a kindergarten classroom, there are so many things that we could be doing; it'd be great to have more than twenty minutes, but we can be teaching emotional regulation skills, mindfulness skills, social competency skills, nothing controversial, nothing that's partisan.

How can kids get along with each other? How can they understand stressors as not always being their fault? Really helping kids know how to handle conflict and ways that are appropriate; it would have a lifetime effect on them—but also financially. One kid with conduct disorder costs $1 to $2 million for taxpayers because their parent is staying home for work. They're going to use the juvenile justice system. They're going to use the healthcare system. They're going to use the educational system in different ways, and we're talking about twenty minutes in kindergarten to avoid some of those outcomes; it makes good humanitarian sense, good financial sense.

JB: How do we jumpstart this and get the attention of policymakers?

MP: I've never met a teacher or school counselor who says they're not desperate for this kind of information. They want to learn, and they want to integrate or get help integrating this. I think the issues are, there's a little bit on the policy side and a little bit on the public side. We've got to get away from the idea that teaching psychological skills is somehow conveying a woke mindset or critical race theory; this is different. I think people are mixing up the terms. You know, we're just talking about conflict resolution, stress management; this has nothing to do with the more partisan kind of debates going on.

JB: No, it has to do with the skills you learn.

MP: That's right.

JB: Just like academics, K–12, and then when you go to college, and you're *really* on your own, how do you handle conflict and stress and taking care of yourself from self-care and resilience issues? If you're not taught that when you're younger, then where are you? One thing I do want to add is so much has happened over the past three years. That's an understatement. And when you think about how, yes, teachers and counselors and everyone in schools are completely overwhelmed, there was no planning to teach on Zoom; it was pretty much like the next day. When you think about why a student is not behaving academically or emotionally in that setting, well, let's look at that student as a whole person. Did they lose someone? Did they lose a parent? Is their parent abusing them or experiencing a job loss? I could fill in a whole list of blanks here, correct?

MP: Absolutely. A number of kids who are grieving the loss of a parent or someone who lived in their household. There are so many factors. One of the parts of the conversation that I wish there was more attention toward is even if we take it away from mental illness, let's take out the people who are suffering so much. They would need a clinical diagnosis, and they might not be able to function on a daily basis in their normal tasks. Let's just look at the skills among the population that does not have a diagnosis right now. We spend so much time and energy teaching people the skills they need to succeed at a craft or a competency to get a job. But everyone knows that if that person is socially incompetent, if they create drama at work, because they're emotionally hot-headed, if they create conflicts, that is taking so much time and energy from the workplace. It's costing money, and it's causing emotional distress for everyone around them. This is the kind of thing that we're also talking about is prevention, by teaching the basic social skills, competency, emotion regulation skills, because hopefully it will prevent the severe mental illness, and of course, that's extremely important. I think helping people see that it's not just to help prevent serious mental illness. These are skills we all need in life. No one is getting hired or promoted if they're horrible on emotional regulation or conflict resolution. These are life skills just as important as teaching math and reading and the ability to critically analyze a reading document—reading comprehension—but that's not the way our system is built right now. We're not built to think about a holistic approach toward child development.

JB: Well, you can also break the cycle. If you're teaching a student to not lash out when things don't go their way, maybe they learned that at home or from someone else, and if you're teaching them how to manage their emotions and to communicate effectively, they'll use that throughout their lifetime. If they don't, they're perpetuating the cycle of verbal and emotional abuse.

MP: And they might even come home from learning it in elementary school and talk with their parents about it and affect their own parents, as well as the next generation. I think you're exactly right; this is a multi-generational strategy, and it's a way that we can really level some systemic inequities. It's a way that we can provide a level playing ground because, let's face it, a lot of people who have some struggles might be because there are struggles going on at home, and it's hard. We can't expect for this to be done in the household.

JB: Right. Everything from food insecurity to loss of a parent, divorce, illness, and more; this can reflect what's going on at home. A lot of times students are saying, "I don't feel heard. I don't feel listened to." People aren't being kind and compassionate, and they are expected to just "go back to the way things were." It's not like that anymore.

MP: Well, here's the problem on the policy end with getting this done. The mental health system that we know of today was created for veterans after World War II. That's when there was a huge influx of money into the U.S. We built the National Institute of Mental Health, the VA system, and so on. And it's built on this one-to-one treatment model where you have a therapist, and you have a patient.

Adults can present all kinds of complex scenarios, but in some cases, an adult can walk in and say I'm feeling depressed, and you can start treatment within that hour for depression. None of this applies for kids. Kids don't walk in and say I'm depressed, and you start treatment. Kids are embedded in systems—a school system, a home system, a community system. Just figuring out what's going on for kids is much more complex. Treating kids is treating the climate—the entire environment or systems in which kids live.

On the policy level, people are saying there's a youth mental health crisis. What do we do? Let's put a little bit more money in the current systems, but that system is built for adults. There's a sense that it would actually cost so much money and it feels too big, especially in the political climate that we're in now, to imagine how do we build an entire new system. But if you look at the Surgeon General Report, calling out youth mental health as a national crisis, it's exactly what that report says. These are systems of embedded influence on kids, and we need a whole new way of addressing this.

JB: The participants of the Mental Health Youth Action Forum went to DC, and they have amazing ideas. Some of them are part of a summer series I put together in July because I want to hear what they have to say, their creativity and ideas. With regards to our mental healthcare system, there needs to be a complete overhaul. There needs to be a needs assessment because they're the customer. I'll use the example of creating a candy bar. I say to you, "Gen Z is going to love this, Mitch," and you ask, "What's in it?" I say, "They're going to love it. I didn't test it on them, but it has kale, broccoli, and carrots." When I do test it on them, they say, "This is garbage." You have to go to the customer and ask, "How are you feeling? What do you want?" I don't have to tell you this.

MP: I would 100 percent agree with you that the model that kids would say they need today is something where mental health is infused into everything because the fact is, we're the ones that still hold on to stigma. The kids don't. They *want* to talk about this. They *do* talk about this. They have multiple online platforms where they do talk about this. *We're the ones* who are the problem. And they would say, "We're happy to do therapy online. We're happy to do it on Twitter, we're happy to do it in peer groups. We don't have a problem talking about this in our classrooms. I think that your point about having this be youth driven is 100 percent correct.

The truth is, they've also grown up in a world where they have lost some in-person interaction. Research that we've been doing in our lab has been demonstrating that, and this is under review right now, but in the hour after they engage in social media use, they actually feel lonelier; they're craving interpersonal interaction. But they're only familiar with a way of doing it that actually ends up backfiring; it makes them feel lonelier rather than happier. I'm not saying that social media is all bad, or that it's the cause for all, but I think it's part of what's going on is that kids are growing up in a world that's different than ours, and it might present some more risks. That's another thing they've inherited, and now they have to live through it. We don't know it; we don't live it in the same way they do.

JB: The lure of the technology is almost like a brainwashing— maybe this word is too strong. We are all so hooked. We're swiping and we're looking at somebody else's life. We don't even know these people. There's such a lure, and we are not present in our own lives, our own relationships.

MP: The part of the brain that develops first in adolescence because our brains don't mature all at once, but little by little, is an area that is filled with dopamine and oxytocin receptors multiplying as we go through puberty. The research is demonstrating that social media activates that particular region of the brain in a way that is pretty similar to the way that we've seen with illegal substances.

We taught a class at UNC Chapel Hill, and we asked undergraduates in the class—we have done this now with four or five hundred undergraduates. We took the DSM criteria for substance dependence disorder, the extent to which you go out of your way to make sure you have access to a substance. You're nervous about times you won't be able to get it. It's interfering with your day. We switched out substance for social media. We literally listed the criteria exactly as it was. The extent to which you know you should stop it but just can't help yourself. Between 80 percent and 100 percent of the kids endorsed every one of those items; this isn't a true diagnosis at this stage but just our ability to use what we know about symptoms of addiction as applied to social media. A remarkably high percentage of kids is saying that. I think your instincts and your take on that is really supported by data now—that we do see the areas of the brain and the kids' responses as indicating this has become an addiction.

JB: So, here we are in a mental health pandemic. How do you think, besides policy change, we are going to get out of it?

MP: What I would love to see happen is that we need to start bringing mental health screening into more of a universal fashion; that could mean anything from at home, just talking about it more openly, but it could also mean that a classroom or a school-based level or a community-based level to do the screenings. We have the instruments, so we know how to do this the same way that we can ask you two or three questions and know whether you're at risk for heart disease. We can do that for mental health too. There's no reason why we shouldn't be doing that, except that many schools that are very interested in doing this when they start hearing how many kids are in need of services. They elect not to do the screenings because they're fearful that then they'll be liable, and there aren't enough providers in the community to help these kids.

We need a multi-pronged approach. Screenings, yes, but also, we need to start taking advantage of lay providers that can be trained to deliver, if not crisis intervention services... at least something until we have more opportunity to bring people to licensed mental health professionals. It's got to be multi-tiered, and once you say that, people quickly throw their hands up and say, "It's too complex. We can't do it." We all bury our heads in the sand again for another decade or two.

JB: Well, it's apathy and not opening a Pandora's box.

MP: Yeah, you're right, but we can do this. Again, I will go back to World War II. We did it. We, as a country, said, "This is important." We built psychology departments on every campus. We trained a huge workforce of clinical counseling and school psychologists. We just need people to stand up and say, "It's time to do that again. This is more important than the other things on the agenda." Our children's health is more important than anything else.

JB: It's upsetting to me when I see reports and data, and when I'm talking to Gen Z, and they're saying all this research and data is great, but what are we doing about it now?

MP: There is a mental health package that's being talked about on the hill. We'll see what happens. There are ways that we're trying to get a much more diverse mental health workforce; that's also so important because we need to have providers that look like and come from the communities where people have needs, and I think right now we have that skewed in ways that are not good.

Young people have made their older counterparts listen on so many factors, and it's not their burden to do it again, but I will say to the older folks, it's ours to listen. And if we hear young people saying that this is important, they're ready to talk about it. They want to talk about mental health. They are suffering. We need to listen to them because it's not a phase; it's not something that all kids go through. It's not something that's just going to pass. When a kid spends six months feeling depression, actually about three months is the most common length of a depressive episode. Three months. That is distorting an entire trajectory of that kid's educational development, their relationship development.

If they spent three months not talking with their friends as often, not going out, not paying attention in school, imagine a small change, and where you're pointed might look very small for the next few steps. But if you carry out how that new direction is going to look five to ten years from now, it's taking you to a place very far from where you would have ended up. I always try to explain to people losing three, six, nine, twelve months to mental illness can have a lifelong consequence. Let's not be shortsighted and think this is just a phase; this can affect a generation.

JB: I have heard Gen Z tell me they want to hear adults share their stories. They want to hear you're depressed too. I feel that they need to hear truths and compassion.

MP: I think I tweeted out once that epidemiological data suggests that 85 percent of humans will experience a DSM diagnosis (Diagnostic and Statistical Manual of Mental Disorders) at some point in their lives. I was like, the jig is up, people! We're all going to experience this at some point. For some people, maybe for years or decades, but for other people, maybe it will be short-lived. There's nothing to hide anymore. Let's all just own up to the fact that yes, this applies to everyone, and there's not a person on earth who has not experienced something already or has not known someone, loved someone, or cared deeply about someone who has not suffered with a mental illness difficulty at this point. We're being so antiquated and foolish. We're looking back to the 1600s where we thought that evil spirits were the cause for mental illness, and it's so silly that our willingness to talk about it is still coming from taboo topics from hundreds of years ago. Let's be modern and recognize that. Come on! If you suffer from mental illness, there's no reason to feel shame or embarrassment about it, any more than if you had caught the flu.

Meet Dr. Raeleen Manjak

DM/OL, ΔMΔ, CPHR
Director of Human Resources, Vernon, British Columbia, Canada

"The pandemic really shone a spotlight on the importance of wellness/well-being, and not just our physical health wellness/well-being but our social, emotional, and mental health."

—Dr. Raeleen Manjak

I met award-winning Director of Human Resources, Dr. Raeleen Manjak, on LinkedIn when she posted an article about employers prioritizing the mental health of their employees. Dr. Manjak is very passionate about mental health initiatives and the importance of kindness and compassion in the workplace.

Janeane Bernstein (JB): When we spoke previously, I had mentioned we were in a mental health crisis prior to March 2020. How do you think we ended up there?

Raeleen Manjak (RM): That's such a compelling question because I think that the pandemic will have significant impacts on people's mental health, but obviously, we were there before that even happened. This is probably the biggest health crisis of our time, and the pandemic has exacerbated what already existed, especially for people who were already experiencing complex mental health or addiction issues. Organizations need to look at the science to show us the way, because our patterns and practices are truly shaped by what we do, not by what we know. In HR, leaders should be looking to create that culture of support for employees once we've emerged from the primary COVID chaos.

I asked Raeleen to share details of her work and her involvement in the mental well-being of her employees.

RM: I'm the Director of Human Resources for the City of Vernon, and we look after all of our employees. This is one of our central service delivery provisions. In addition to the typical types of human resource functions, for example, talent acquisition and retention, occupational health and safety, payroll, and benefits, learning and development, and labor relations, we also created a new position called Employee Care Coordinator. This emerged prior to COVID, and we're so thankful that we have this embedded in place because we were better able to care for our people.

JB: It sounds like a preventative measure.

RM: It is. It's really about providing moments of support and resilience for people because you can share resilience; it's a shared competency to really be there for them as they experience changes or perhaps opportunities within their current work cycle. Before the pandemic, we had actually provided lunch and learns for our employee groups in all of the areas of mental well-being, so stress, anxiety, burnout, grief, depression. We worked through all of those items.

We also held an annual health and wellness fair for our entire target population so that folks can come in and see what types of health and wellness/well-being supports are available in our community. All of the providers came to our recreation complex, and they set up their booths and then our employees visited all of the booths, and they had a great lunch. We offer plenary sessions on topics of key interest, and we just really want to be there to support people in their whole selves. Because when you bring your whole self to work, it's really a place of belonging, and we want to do whatever we can to make sure that that exists.

JB: One of the things I've been hearing a lot in my conversations is that people want to feel heard; they want to connect in a kind way, where people are compassionate and empathetic, and this is the time to do it.

RM: Well, I think the pandemic really shone a spotlight on the importance of wellness/well-being, and not just our physical health wellness/well-being but our social, emotional, and mental health, all of the dimensions. In the wake of uncertainty and physical distancing, we saw many companies making that critical shift to meaningful connection and supporting their people's mental wellness/well-being in new ways, including regular formal and informal check-ins, modeling healthy leadership behaviors, increasing mental health education and benefits.

I'd say that the discussion on mental health has long been overdue. It's taken the pandemic to clearly see that being healthy is so much more than just being physically well because health exists on a spectrum. And we don't really understand or apply this to mental health in our discussions or beliefs. And so, as quickly as the pandemic really required that shift, so has the emerging and evolving definition of what mental health and wellness/well-being really means. It's an opportunity for people like you and me, and the work that you do is just extraordinary, which is really inextricably linked across all dimensions of health.

I've been doing quite a bit of research lately because I really want to try to bring in all kinds of opportunities for our employees. And one of the things that recently has come up is what researchers are calling this psychological immune system. This is a collection of those cognitive abilities that we all have that enable us to make the best even in a worst situation scenario.

The pandemic has actually been a test of that across the globe. The research is offering what appears to be that we have a more robust function than we ever would have guessed because when those familiar sources of enjoyment kind of all evaporated in the spring of 2020, we really got creative. We participated in drive-by birthday parties and mutual assistance groups and virtual cocktail evenings with old friends and nightly...

JB: Sourdough bread baking!

RM: Sourdough bread baking if you've never baked bread before! All of those things help us reweave our social tapestry. We're recreating our web of connections. I think that it's really important that we recognize that those broad trends don't erase the real struggles. Some people had immense pain, overwhelming loss, financial hardships, and that's not all, but there was astonishing resilience exhibited in the face of sudden changes brought on by the pandemic. I would say it holds its own lessons. We've learned that people can handle temporary changes to their lifestyle, like working from home, giving up travel, or going into isolation better than what we seemed to assume prior to the pandemic.

JB: I think of all the factors that are contributing to the mental health pandemic: the anxiety and depression, suicide rates, abuse, job loss, food insecurity, college students that can't go home, and they're sleeping in their cars—there are so many scenarios—make me realize, schools, businesses, people in general need to find ways to be compassionate and rethink the way they were doing things.

RM: New studies are coming out all the time from a global research perspective offering that we are starting to come out of those situations where we are anxious, depressed, and traumatized. Trauma is a significant factor here. However, it is not a generalized statement. Studies find that stress and anxiety fuel poor sleep, fatigue issues, and start to create a cycle around unwellness. The more we lay awake at night, rehashing the worries (that we have no control over), the worse our mental health becomes. You mentioned domestic violence; it is increasing worldwide. Preliminary results from surveys that have been conducted scientifically confirmed this trend. Domestic violence cases for people who were already experiencing some type of it have gotten worse in nearly 60 percent of the cases, and it really comes down to a variety of factors: people spending more time at home, potentially with abusive partners, unemployment, other financial stressors causing conflict. Shelters are shutting their doors. Police are being discouraged from making arrests.

Needless to say, the threat of abuse truly is compounding the stress, anxiety, and fear that many people were already experiencing well before the pandemic arrived. I would say that the effects depend on personality, lifestyle, and demographics, and I don't think we can forget any of those indicators. Personality influences how we fare in tough times. Two related traits that really seem to rise are our ability to tolerate uncertainty and our ability to tolerate distress. It's really hard for anyone to struggle or face the unknown. Some people are less comfortable with it than others and right now. It's those people who may be ruminating a little more, feeling more afraid, or experiencing more depression, anxiety, or even PTSD. People with poor health or chronic disease tend to have higher symptoms of stress, anxiety, depression, and PTSD. That's what the studies are finding. And these people may be at greater risk for COVID. You talk about education. Let's talk about income and education because both of those things matter. The less stable your income and the less educated you are, studies suggest the more anxiety, depression, and stress you may actually experience. With the pandemic threatening the economy, it has affected financial futures, but the situation, really, Janeane, is worse for those who were already struggling.

We are not all in the same boat at all. And for those who are disadvantaged, the effects are further compounded. These groups are suffering disproportionately under the pandemic. All of those inequities we've discussed create mental health problems that are even more aggravated by reducing unequal access to service. And discrimination—we see it rising within communities right across the globe. As you know, medical and healthcare workers have taken on that urgent task of continued care of patients, putting themselves at risk. Some positions have transitioned to remote work or hybrid work.

JB: Or they left.

RM: Correct.

JB: I'm thinking about the exodus of teachers, healthcare workers, and so on. No one was prepared for a pandemic.

RM: No. It created a situation where sometimes we had to precariously juggle work, childcare, and eldercare. Working in an office may have seemed to increase risk. We found in our City of Vernon that our vigilance to safety layers provided us opportunities where we didn't have an organizational outbreak. The research notes that there were more stressors from those who were impacted and were working from home. In our city, we didn't shut our doors at all from the onset of the pandemic. We just increased our safety layers immediately. We put all our healthcare protocols in place, and we were hyper-vigilant in our practices. And I can say for myself, this connection to my working relationships and my colleagues, this shared community that we had and the feeling that we were all working together toward an outcome, absolutely assisted in coping with the stress of the pandemic and finding that sense of control at times when there was little control or perhaps even a feeling of helplessness.

I consider you part of my community, this community of practice who are elevating these topics that were once only whispered. We have to stop doing that. We need to bring it into the light, and we have to remove the stigma around this, so that mental health is talked about the same way that a physical health issue is. When somebody breaks an arm, you can actually see that. Somebody's having a need to have a mental health moment where they need to go home and they need to do all of the things to take care of themselves—to see their counselors, to talk to people that are part of their care team. Take moments for that critical type of reflection and self-care. That is exactly the same way we need to treat mental wellness/well-being—the same way as we would treat a physical health issue.

JB: Any advice on how we can be better and do better to one another?

RM: Great question. I think we need to just start. One thing for certain is that we continue to live in uncertain times. I don't think that that's going to change for quite some time. People across the globe are experiencing challenges, and we are collectively coping in this worldwide event. The results aren't uplifting, but they aren't surprising either. We're suffering, and some of us are suffering worse than others. You don't have to have lost a job or a loved one to be affected. Humans are complex, and so are emotional responses.

When this all started, we learned how the virus spreads, how to wash our hands, how to wear a mask, how to physically distance. I'm sure that if we didn't know what two meters or six feet looked like pre-pandemic, we certainly do now. So, we have lessons to learn about what happens to mental health in a crisis like this, and we need to find ways to address that.

I would say that part of that shift is really to recognize, across all of the dimensions of health and wellness/well-being, what may be trending in 2022 and beyond.

There's a variety of trends that support mental health and wellness/well-being, including intellectual and financial wellness/well-being, mental health programming. You talk a little bit about education, access to education, support for people who are going through that, virtual and telehealth care, the improved emphasis on work and life integration. I'd really like to talk about that; it's not about balance, right? I mean, people say, well, I need more "work-life balance." What is that? I've never really figured out what that means.

For me, it's about integration. Sometimes my work takes a little more time. Sometimes my life takes a little more time. So how do I integrate those two spheres so that I can create a sense of well-being inside my own body? We can't look around and not see what the effect that social media use has on everything, both from a positive aspect and a negative aspect. Learning and development opportunities around trauma-informed care is so important. There's so much information out there, and if you do one thing, read about what trauma informed care is because if we can't self-improve our way out of pain and difficulty, we can certainly help someone else do that.

We're going through a trauma, Janeane. This is a trauma and a major stressor on a global scale. This is one of the times when life really is harder by a little bit, or by a lot, depending on your situation. And to feel bad about it is part of being human. And right now, that's something that many of us need to face, even as we work to feel better. We need to stay connected, and we need to help others. For me, I did a bit of research. UC Berkeley has a great class in the science of happiness. And they talk about what that means. They go all the way back to the beginning of the great philosophers, Confucius, Plato, Aristotle, and they start talking about what that means. And that common thread that is pulled all the way back from the beginning of time is really connection.

JB: The power of connection.

RM: Yes, absolutely. So yes, connect to one person. Connect to two or three key people in your life. It doesn't have to be a circle of a hundred, but you should be connected to somebody. And if you feel like you're isolated and there's just nobody out there, there is somebody out there. There is somebody. Reach out.

JB: I read a lot of research the past year about the power of connecting intergenerationally, such as college students and retirees. Let's say somebody is in a retirement home, and they're secluded for safety—isolated from COVID. They're not seeing anyone, and they're prone to depression. They might feel their life doesn't have value. They're not engaged. But when you connect them with college students, there have been different studies and research about how you can light up different generations. I'm so interested in creating projects that foster connection.

RM: I think if we each took a moment and realized that this pandemic is something new to us. But the impact that it has had is not new to us. Going through the Great Depression, going through recessions, going through a World War, going through the impact of what the Holocaust, all of these life lessons create opportunities for great encyclopedias of experience. If we can put our younger generation in contact with people who have all of that depth, lived experience on coping strategies around what they did at a time when they couldn't pick up a phone and just look something up on Google. I think it would create just a depth of wonder for people and an opportunity to, like you say, elevate and cross generationally impact on more than one level.

I think we need to remember that as human beings, we're not passive victims of change. We can be active stewards of our own well-being, and we should be empowered to make those changes in our community or country in our global society as we support the individuals and communities that have been the hardest hit. And we need to be vigilant in that connection and the protection of connection because it's really easy to just say no, I'm not going to do that. Because it's the little things that we do. It's those tiny moments, those microseconds, those moments in time when you turn around to somebody in the grocery store line and you say, "How are you doing today?" and you have a smile on your face. Or you see somebody who looks like something's going on and you just stop for a moment, and you have a touchpoint with them. Because that is a form of recognition.

And if people feel that they're being seen, it makes all the difference in the world. And for me, it's the little things. It's the daily routines. I'm a meditator, so even if I only have ten minutes, I find a way to really just settle into that practice, to be gracious and give gratitude about all of the gifts in my life. And it's the way we deal with our emotions in our care for others. That will remind us that our actions make a difference every single day.

JB: Well, it's true if you look for the moments; they can be micro-moments. I'll give you an example. I was going to return some things to the grocery store. I had a loaf of bread, and as I'm driving down the street, I see this woman holding up a sign saying she was experiencing homelessness, and she's "hungry and anything would help." I'm in the middle lane. There's a car blocking my view of her. So, I rolled down my window and yelled, "Are you hungry?!" And she responded back, "Yes!" So, I made my way over to her and handed her this big loaf of bread, and she was so happy. As I drove away, she stood there cradling her bread. All I did was look around my car to see what I could give her. That's how I believe we should live our lives—by asking ourselves, "What can I do?" Let's look up from our phones, focus on someone else, and be thoughtful.

Meet Dr. Bryan E. Robinson

Psychotherapist
Licensed Marriage and Family Therapist
Licensed Clinical Mental Health Counselor
Co-founder and Chief Architect, ComfortZones Digital

"A lot of the younger people who were working are saying you're not going to treat me this way; A lot of the younger folks are saying I'm not going to sacrifice myself. I want to work at a place that cares about me, that treats me with respect—that is more important than the money and the benefits. People are tired of the Dark Age way corporate America has been treating employees and they're not going to do it anymore, and that's a huge result of the pandemic."

—Bryan E. Robinson, PhD

I met Dr. Bryan Robinson several years ago when I interviewed him about his book, *#CHILL—Turn Off Your Job and Turn On Your Life*.

Dr. Robinson began our conversation by sharing how the pandemic impacted his professional life as a psychotherapist and the lives of his patients.

Bryan Robinson (BR): Like most therapists, I was doing all digital virtual therapy, but it's been sobering to see how many people are struggling with mental health issues, not just here, but all over the world, and the amount of burnout that's occurring is just through the roof. People have been suffering, and some still are just with the isolation and starting to question, "Who am I and do I want to keep doing this?" Because life's so short and motivates potential questions coming up for people, which is why we have the great resignation. Four million people in February left their jobs. It's been a huge transformation, personally, workwise, and socially.

It's affecting everybody, but especially the younger generation today is really having trouble. One of the things that I always come back to is self-care—but a different kind of self-care. You know, we think of self-care as most people think of exercising—taking a bubble bath, eating well, getting good sleep. Those are all critical and are the foundation, but lately, I've started taking it a step further because we're dealing with such challenging issues. I talk about radical self-care. The word radical to me is a different thing for each person. But when I say radical self-care, a lot of people think self-care is selfish or narcissistic. It is not. Self-care and self-compassion are one of the most important things we can do for ourselves, because nobody on this planet can do that for Janeane or Bryan, except Janeane and Bryan.

And it's like, that airplane metaphor—if the oxygen masks dislodge, you better put it on first. It's a good way to think about it because that didn't sound so selfish. But if we talk about somebody wanting me to do something and I feel guilty because I need to rest, but I'm going to go ahead and do it anyway—that's not okay. It's okay to say no, and it's okay to put yourself first if you're already stressed and burned out, and a lot of people don't know that. It seems like a simple concept. But I think we need to get back to the way we build these blocks whether it's community, nationally, or internationally—we need to start with ourselves first. If I'm in good shape, mentally and physically, then I can help other people, and I can help change things in my own corner of the world.

I keep up with neuroscience. I'm not a neuroscientist, but I'm fascinated by the mind–body connection. Historically, people have thought that was kind of "woo woo," you know, strange. What does the body have to do with the mind? But I want to mention a recent study I read just as an example. The neuroscientists studied two groups of people, one of which practice self-compassion. They treated themselves like they would their best friend or a family member. They did nice things for themselves. Those folks, compared to the other group who did not practice self-compassion, had lower cardiovascular risk. Now, they measured that by measuring the linings of the blood vessels in both groups, and they found less plaque and thinner linings of people who practice self-compassion. So, whatever we think and feel will find its way into the body. That's just one example. But treating ourselves with care and love is a healthy thing to do; it's not a narcissistic thing.

JB: Yes, and when you think about all the factors that compounded stress the past few years, more reason to focus on self-care.

BR: Yes, and that includes the way we talk to ourselves. When I see clients, we all use the word *should* and we all use the word *must*. And we all use the words *I have to*, but when you really take a breath and step back, those words are oppressive. And we don't realize what we're doing to our internal nervous system. In fact, a lot of psychologists use terms like *should-y* thinking or *must-urbation* to help people remember when you're using those words, you're stressing yourself out because you're imposing pressure on yourself, and that's just a micro-change, a micro-adjustment. If you catch yourself when you're "should-ing" on yourself or "must-erbaiting," and say, I *get* to do my homework or I *get* to go for that job interview or I *get* to help my friend or I *get* to go to work. Instead of I *have to* or *must*, it makes a big difference in and what gets translated into our bodies.

JB: I started going to therapy a year ago, and there's a lot of patterns from negative thoughts that came from negative people when I was younger. I just kept those stories on repeat, those opinions on repeat, and they don't add any value to my life.

BR: That is right. They extract the value. Scientists talk about a negativity bias. So, we do have a hardwired predisposition to look at the negative for survival. We all have that; that's just part of what Mother Nature gave us because she wanted us to survive. Knowing that there are times if you're walking from your office into the dark parking garage, you want to pay attention, especially nowadays with what's going on in the news. However, you also want to be vigilant that there are times when we may be looking at the negative side of something, when in fact it doesn't relate to survival. Could be a relationship or our job or our parenting. It's important to ask yourself, "How am I looking at this situation?" Take a breath and step back and see if you can look at it in a different way. I call it expanding your perspective.

Dr. Robinson went on to share his thoughts on what can be done in schools and businesses to facilitate positive change and move us out of the mental health pandemic.

BR: I do think it starts with each one of us individually in our own little corner of the world, but more globally in schools and nationwide, it involves education. I think the first thing that needs to happen, and this is happening actually, is we need people to know that mental health is no different from physical health, but we treat it differently. There's a stigma to it. So, removing the stigma of mental health, and people understanding that if you have a mental illness, that's no different really than having a headache or a shoulder that needs surgery or whatever. Naomi Osaka was forced to confront the press when she was struggling with anxiety and depression, and they fined her $15,000. Then they said either you meet the press and deal with this or you're out of here. Well, think about that. Now, if she had a physical injury, they wouldn't have required that. She was one of the top tennis players. When she stepped back and said, "I am not going to do this," she was scorned by people. That is a great example of how we have to rethink mental health.

If you got a broken leg and you have a cast and you need time off, you need people to help you. We need to have that same outlook with mental illness or mental health. We don't, and that's unfortunate. So, I think that's where it all begins, and I think that it should begin with schools. I think we should be talking about mental health and mental illness and what it really is. People are scared of it. They think it's strange or weird, but it isn't. We're all in the same boat. You and I were just talking about this. We're all struggling with something—every single person reading right now. You're struggling with something, and that makes you normal. We're all in the same boat. We just don't talk about it because we're afraid somebody will think we're strange or we'll be judged, and that is what we need to get over.

I see so many kids who go off to college unprepared for the stress; it's that transition into being more of an adult because you're away from home. They are not prepared for the stress, and that's when some people end up with depression, anxiety, anorexia, eating disorders, substance abuse. Trying to cope with stress because they don't have the armor, the equipment to do it.

JB: I really do feel that policies need to be put into place in schools. It starts in schools and then businesses. Not every age group will be comfortable saying, "I'm going to take a mental health day." I know, talking to perhaps Gen Z, some tend to be more comfortable opening up and saying, "I'm taking a mental health day." And somebody says, "Why did you take a picture of yourself at the beach?" That was your mental health day. Sitting with a book on the beach. I mean, it's really no one's business. This is how you're spending your mental health day, but we do need to normalize it.

BR: Yes. And the way we're talking more about in business normalizing mental health days and more companies are starting to offer that instead of even calling it a sick day— call it a Mental Health Day. I like the idea of flipping and calling it "have more green time to off balance my screen time."

Most of us are thinking about the next thing we were going to do or what we didn't do right yesterday or what's upcoming. We might be worried about a test or an exam or a presentation we have to give. But what we have found in the research is if I can start to be aware, because I'm already thinking about tomorrow and I'm not in the right now. When we can be more in the right now, we call it mindfulness. A powerful tool to learn when our mind starts wandering is to bring it back with love and compassion and just notice in this moment what's going on. Listen to the sounds around you for just a few minutes or notice the colors or the sky or the trees. That is a micro-chiller. You will notice in one minute you're calmer if you do it for five minutes. You notice that even more and if you have a practice, because it builds up over time. So, what you're feeling inside overshadows or gives you more power to deal with whatever is looming on the horizon.

I wrapped up our conversation by asking Dr. Robinson if he has found learning moments in the pandemic, such as the realization that society was running at such a fast speed, focusing on individual wants and behaviors, and not being thoughtful to others.

BR: Yes, I remember here in Asheville, when the pandemic first started, and people were quarantining, I noticed how people were allowing other people to get in front of them. I think nationally, we even found that there were fewer mass shootings for a lot of reasons. I was at Starbucks, at the drive-thru, and started to pay and the woman said the person in front of us already paid for your coffee, which seems like an insignificant thing, but it isn't. It's indicative of a feeling—a mood. When I look at what's going on in Ukraine now, it seems like when we have tragedy, sometimes there's a lining in that. When we look at the spirit of the people in Ukraine,

I keep thinking, how can we build that here again in our country? I think it starts with those small little gestures of love.

Meet Kelechi Ubozoh

Mental Health Consultant, Advocate, Writer, Published Author

"We don't have robust conversations about mental health and there is a lot of stigma in different school communities about what can be shared and not shared. I think it depends on your school culture, but there has been a reluctance to have these conversations, because they don't want to open the door for things, but the door has already been open."

—Kelechi Ubozoh

Kelechi Ubozoh and I met when she was a guest on my show in 2021. I was extremely moved by her mental health advocacy work and other impactful initiatives.

Janeane Bernstein (JB): How do you think we got to the place of being in a mental health crisis before the pandemic?

Kelechi Ubozoh (KU): That's such a good question. I guess it depends on who you are or where you sit, but on one hand, on the more personal and emotional level, a lot of us have not paid attention to our needs. A lot of us have not listened to our boundaries. A lot of us have been holding things for years, just working and grinding and surviving. And I know there was a lot of tension and upset with the 2016 elections. I feel like there was a huge split between our country, and this "us versus them" fallout. So, this energy of having us feel split as a collective and then combining that with at our systemic challenges, heightened violence, increased visibility of racism and discrimination, climate crises, and if you live in California, the specific experience we've had around fires and the traumatic losses from those fires and how they've only gotten worse. There is so much more, but when I think about it, we've had so many crises bubbling up, whether they be political, climate, racialized; there has been just a breakdown in how we connect with each other. And I think that was some of this was the precursor to the explosion that occurred in March of 2020. I wouldn't say that it has ended, but things just built and built and built more.

JB: Like a volcano.

KU: Yeah, absolutely. That's a great analogy. I can see that metaphor. So yes, things built like a volcano, and it erupted.

JB: And then some of the factors contributing to the pandemic—over forty million people out of work. What else do you think contributed to the pandemic that we're in?

KU: Well, even just going back to the fact that we've been isolated, people were really looking forward to graduations and weddings and connecting with people in person. A lot of us took that for granted—I know I did. I never thought we would be in a situation where we could not touch people, hold people, and be in people's presence for an extended period of time. For many, the impact of this isolation has had such a devasting effect on our mental health and well-being.

JB: There was the horrible death of George Floyd and other events that were happening before and during the pandemic. It just fueled the fire and raised a lot of different issues. Do you feel there are a lot of big learning moments for us as humans?

KU: So many people called 2020 a "racial reckoning" because it was the first time *globally* folks were listening to the words "Black Lives Matter." And I must underscore that Black Lives Matter is not a new movement by any means; it started in 2013. But I believe the public killing of George Floyd by law enforcement could not be ignored. People could not look away, and I believe folks were able to look and listen and sit with this pain, this violence, this injustice and finally say, this is wrong. We know that Black and Brown folks are killed for existing, playing in the park (Tamir Rice), breathing, walking home from a store (Trayvon Martin), sleeping in their beds (Breonna Taylor), or jogging (Ahmaud Arbery). This isn't new. But I think people were forced to look because they had nowhere else to go. There were no distractions. You were in your house. And yet, not everyone was home. We have to remember all the people who didn't get to be in their houses because they were taking care of everyone else, but a lot of folks were at home.

And you did have those big opportunities to really look at racialized violence in the United States, including the rise in hate crimes against the Asian American and Pacific Islander communities during the pandemic. We got to have conversations that people weren't having before across different backgrounds, racial identities, and ethnicities. And yes, some of what happened was performative and short-lived, but some of those conversations and that work continues.

We also started having the mental health conversation, even if weren't using the words "mental health." People were way more open to having conversations about the impact of isolation, feeling depressed and depleted, and the importance of self-care and healing. Even if the words were different, the need to look inward was really felt communally. Folks started looking for therapists and providers to support them as they're dealing with their grief of losing loved ones, sitting with the impact of the racialized violence impacting their communities, and navigating being isolated.

I also think people began to really to feel more connected to what they deserve. Because for a lot of people who were working in jobs that never took a break, they just shifted from, "Okay, we're not in person and working from home" and now you *really* have no break. You're at home all day. And there's no boundaries, so folks left jobs that weren't serving them in droves. A lot of people are like, "I'm not called to do this anymore. This isn't worth this. I'm not going to do this work." Meanwhile, other folks were losing their jobs. So, there was a big tension of scrambling to find anything, and a big feeling of "I don't want to be where I am."

I don't know that people immediately quit at the beginning, but as the pandemic went on, people left. A mass exodus of people left big expensive cities, really feeling like, "Oh, this cost of living never made sense, but it certainly doesn't make sense now. What would it be like to be somewhere with spaciousness, actual land, or be in on the water or to be with/ near your family?" I think there was almost a reckoning of what's going on in the external world of witnessing so much death, police brutality, extreme poverty, and all these huge moments and then there was an internal reckoning of what do I deserve? What do I want? What does my family need? Where do we need to be right now? Is this job serving my mental health? And folks made some really big changes, huge changes.

JB: The *New York Times* published an article about how moms were hit really hard in the pandemic. They're juggling their whole life under one roof, and the kids are home, and there is an incredible amount of stress, and menopausal women are leaving work, teachers, nurses, and so on. Everyone is bailing.

KU: Yes, everyone is bailing. And it's no wonder, especially if the conditions weren't good before the pandemic. And then you have this massive global pandemic, world shutdown—a meltdown, truly—and all the systemic holes that were never fixed or received attention are just screaming. And folks do not feel supported. I think we all talked about how much we really appreciate teachers because parents became teachers in a large way while teachers were still trying to handle things. They never stopped doing their work. But then, after all of this "appreciation," have they been supported? Has anything programmatically or systemically changed for them? We heard much messaging "appreciating these frontline staff." Thank you, nurses, thank you doctors, thank you healthcare workers, thank you teachers/educators, thank you truck drivers, cashiers, and agricultural workers, thank you all essential workers. We heard all those platitudes, but when did you change any policies to give folks days off, alleviate their stress, give them extra pay? What is the lesson we should learn for how to protect the folks who are out there during a global crisis, so we don't see these huge gaps in the workforce?

What is your plan? What is your plan for your family? What is your plan for your work? How are you supporting that frontline staff who are going to get burned out? What are you doing to take care of them? Because they're burned out, and now they're gone, and we have this huge void. So, I think there are lessons learned on how we treat these folks that we call our heroes, and what are we doing to actually support these heroes?

JB: That's an excellent point. I feel like there was no infrastructure before. And teachers have to meet certain academic goals, and they don't have time, or they're not also trained properly to be able to be a detective when they see their A student is now failing. They might not have the bandwidth to say, wait a minute, is there something going on at home? Could it be abuse? Could it be lack of food, lack of X, Y and Z? I think the priorities must shift. The real priority is mental health because if you don't have your mental health as a kid, where are you as an adult?

KU: Absolutely. I think that folks have become mental health providers without ever being trained as mental health providers because they are part of those safety nets. If you think of any system, even an ecosystem, what is someone's connection to their environment? Who are those trusted people that they can connect to? For example, say you have a teacher you really like, and you feel close to them, and you share some personal things with them. If we're not preparing teachers to receive all of that emotional expression, and just focusing on making sure these kids pass XYZ for a test because those school grades determine their school's funding *(which I have such strong feelings about teaching for tests as opposed to nurturing and growing humans to be successful)* what capacity do teachers actually have?

And then the conversations about mental health in school. We don't have robust conversations about mental health, and there is a lot of stigma in different school communities about what can be shared and not shared. I think it depends on your school culture, but there has been a reluctance to have these conversations because they don't want to open the door for things, but the door has already been open.

We could direct folks and have them have coping strategies, really understand what's happening when big emotions are happening in their bodies, what a crisis might look like because we are having a youth mental health crisis that is unprecedented. Unprecedented; it is everywhere. Researchers and clinicians are documenting that we're having higher suicide rates for young, young people—we're talking about nine-year-olds, young kids! These are children, and not talking about it doesn't change the fact that it's happening, and saying, "Oh, well, we don't have time to have that in our course catalog" doesn't change the fact that it needs to happen. If not school, then where? I believe space needs for it to happen so educators are supported and don't feel overwhelmed with "one more thing" they have to do. I really believe that it has to be in school.

JB: I do too. I feel that people need to be kinder and more compassionate and good listeners. I have been saying to students, if you can't talk to your parents, find someone you can talk to—find a coach, a mentor, a teacher, a peer, anyone to open up.

KU: Absolutely.

JB: I like that you said this should be a policy issue, because not only schools but really any business. I think there has to be a restructuring because of what is going on. And you talk about "the door's open." I can imagine a line of people kind of in line peeking, going, "Is anybody on the other end listening?"

KU: That is a brilliant observation and conversation because I literally just did this mental health report for racially diverse communities, speaking to community-based organizations who have been providing support like food banks or arts programming and having spaces to connect with each other around whatever is going on in your life, like managing stress and so on. Now, these local organizations have now become de facto emergency rooms for people because communities trust them. But then there's not enough of them. They don't have enough staff because they were never properly funded in the first place, managing burnout and turnover. And so what this pandemic has shown is that we've increased the mental health need, but we have not increased the amount of people to meet the need. And we need to increase the infrastructure and support so that people can do that work and stay in the work as well.

The good news is that people are feeling more comfortable asking for help, and that not so great news is that they are ready to ask for help because they are really struggling and saying, "Okay, fine. I'm ready to have this conversation I never thought I'd have." There has to be something there to meet them and then there isn't enough. And if we overly rely on mental health providers, then we're going to be in trouble because they're burning out too (and there aren't enough of them and long waits to get in). So, this is a conversation for all of us. How can we all be better listeners? How can we all be better prepared to support each other? And that's the humanity piece, not "I'm going to delegate this to someone else, but instead I'm seeing you and I'm going to sit with your pain. I don't have to have your answer, but maybe I can just sit with you and connect." I mean, I think everyone has a role to play. And I think that's really important to remember and observe.

I think sometimes when you're struggling yourself, and yes, you do need to pour back into yourself, but sometimes when you just do something so that you feel small and someone feels gratitude, it totally changes the entire day. I think people think they have to do these huge sweeping efforts to connect. And it's like, "Oh, I'll take these donuts here." Oh, I'm going to be kind to this person because like I literally saw a sign yesterday where it said, "Please don't yell at our staff." And I was just like, wow, you have to put a sign up because people are yelling at your staff? So, no matter how long it takes for my order to come out, I'm going to say, "Thank you so much. How are you?" You know, have a conversation with them.

Be human. People need that connection, that kindness. We're all tired and frustrated. Connection is key. Doing meaningful things that are for other folks is helpful, and it reminds you that you care about people, and you should care about yourself as well. People need to have these conversations, and we need to continue to talk about this.

Meet Dido Balla

Head of Education – MindUP™ | The Goldie Hawn Foundation

"I think it's the perfect opportunity of sitting there for two years to teach kids to understand themselves, to teach emotional intelligence and to make sure that since nobody controls the things that happen to us, at least we can work on controlling what we do with our inside, so a better version can show up to face whatever we don't control, such as a pandemic."

—Dido Balla

I reached out to Dido Balla when I read an article featuring actress, producer, and author Goldie Hawn and her foundation, MindUP™.

Dido and I met before this conversation, and I was moved by his personal and professional journey. I invited him to share his tremendous insight into the mental health of today's youth.

I began by asking Dido to describe what life was like growing up in Cameroon, located in West Central Africa, and whether any childhood struggles shaped his resilience skills as an adult.

> **Dido Balla (DB)**: Things were great because in my mind, I had a normal childhood. It's only when you step back and compare and go back and wonder why this was happening this year [that you realize] things were not great. But for me, things were challenging. I grew up in Cameroon. My parents were renting a small house when I was born. A big dream of theirs was to buy some land and build a house because it would save money. And unfortunately, we couldn't afford to finish building the house. We moved into the house and slowly finished it as we were living there because it was more economical. So, no water. I had to walk long distances to fetch water. We had to add electricity, but for me, that was normal. I thought that's what all kids around the world did.

> **Janeane Bernstein (JB)**: Do you feel like those experiences built resilience skills from an early age?

> **DB**: When I think about my childhood and what I've been through in my life, absolutely. I'm thirty-five, and I was born in Cameroon. I lived in Ethiopia, Nigeria, and Ghana. After all of that, living here is not easy or perfect, but I've experienced things that make me feel like I have some perspective. I am able to have a little more resilience and perspective taking things from those experiences.

Here are Dido's thoughts on the escalation of the mental health crisis, his experiences as a classroom teacher, and lessons learned over the past few years.

DB: The crisis was always there. In fact, I am curious to know what the difference is between the mental health crisis and mental health pandemic. Back when I was in the classroom teaching in 2011, 2012, it was obvious to me that as a country and as youth, we weren't okay. When I started working with MindUP™ and training teachers, it only confirmed that around the country, the youth were dealing with mental health issues; they did not have the tools to regulate, to take care of themselves. It was a little harder to convince adults that this was important. The pandemic forced the world to take a moment. In a society where being on the go is valued, appreciated, and encouraged, being busy is like a badge of honor. In a world where that's the norm, not being able to travel, sitting at home with your own thoughts, your own life forced everybody else, you realize that we haven't been okay for a long time. More and more folks became open to exploring options to do something about it.

JB: I think about the millions and millions of people who lost jobs, the amount of anxiety and depression, suicide, fill in the blank, everything happened. There are so many factors that contributed to the mental health epidemic. And as you said, we were already in this mental health crisis. I'm really hoping that mental health becomes a priority in the curriculum.

DB: Yes, and that's one of my dreams, that we have a curriculum that focuses on neuroscience, mindful awareness, positive psychology, and social emotional learning. And it's a curriculum that's part of a way of life. That means that not only do you have the tools and the content to easily integrate these lessons in your everyday teaching as an educator, but really, this is just the foundation that you need to hopefully shift your mindset throughout life in general and start to look at life with a perspective of how that affects your brain. How is it that I am going to be affected by the fact that in the morning when I wake up, I grab my cell phone? In five minutes, I download all the negative news that happened around the globe. It affects my brain, and that also affects my day.

Because if I start my day that way, of course, when I'm driving to work and somebody cuts me off, I'm already angry, and then that exacerbates my experience. Add to that the collective trauma—wars around the world, poverty— and then of course, we think about minoritized populations, especially—they were already going through a lot even before the pandemic. So yes, we should make it part of teaching but also a part of a new mindset. Just look at the world through a lens of mental health. Who can only benefit from that?

JB: Yes. We have to shift our priorities. I know a lot of parents who want their kids to do well and get into a great college. But long term, let's say they get into a great college, but their mental health is really suffering. What's going to happen when they go to college? They're not going to be able to function, and they're probably going to crash. As you said, you're teaching these life skills that will carry through youth and adulthood. As students get older and face life's ups and downs, those are important life skills, and what really matters is your mental health.

DB: Yeah, it seems to me that the model that we have in our society when it comes to pushing kids to achieve is assuming that the more you achieve, the better school you go into, the higher your grades are, somehow correlate to how happy and fulfilled you will be in life. But that's just not true. The pressure to do the best that you can at school, designed to assign value based on grades, for example, and then students start to attach their inherent value to the grades they get. That's when you start having low self-esteem because a D in math makes you feel like you have already failed life.

You are told that the only way to do well is to increase those grades or graduate from high school. So, you feel that the kids who were doing that are better than you. Somehow you feel as if once you graduate, something great will happen. But then as soon as you graduate, you realize that college is just the beginning of more stress. You're told that if you do well in college or go to the best college and then graduate, then you will get to some sort of happiness or fulfillment. Then you get to college and finish, and then you realize that finding a job is very difficult. Then you find the first job, and you're not happy. The truth is, what you need to do is work on yourself right now from within if your mental health is not okay.

Everything that you experience is through the lens of that person who has low self-esteem, who has not yet been in touch with their emotions, doesn't know how to self-regulate, doesn't know exactly what makes them come alive, and who is just following a path created by other people. Unfortunately, I get to meet those kids when they're adults, and they tell me exactly that; they were on a rat race. They thought that they would find fulfillment and happiness and health when they achieved XYZ. But, of course, now we all know that the younger you can start, like looking into yourself and getting in touch with your mental health and learning how to understand yourself, how to regulate to survive, to seek help, the better you all want to be at achieving all those other things that parents and educators care about.

That's why I put it on the adults because if kids believe that their worth is attached to grades, it's because along the way, enough adults created an environment around them where they were getting attention and validation only when the performance was to a certain degree based on grades. I am not shocked that those students are surprised. We just need more adults to share this message. And one more thing about the pandemic—when schools stopped, we had to redesign, reimagine school virtually or a hybrid model. Many states cancelled the standardized exams that kids take to graduate, and many schools said grades don't really matter right now. If the pandemic allowed them to say that, why is it that it took a pandemic to say that, first of all? If you remove the grades, then the question is what do we do with our time? What are we teaching?

I think it's the perfect opportunity of sitting there for two years to teach kids to understand themselves, to teach emotional intelligence, and make sure that since nobody controls the things that happen to us, at least we can work on controlling what we do with our inside, so a better version can show up to face whatever we don't control, such as a pandemic.

JB: Yes. I want to add something to what you just said because I believe we also have to rethink assessing students' knowledge. Let's say someone is a bad test taker, as was I. Giving students an opportunity to show their knowledge and skills in another way is really powerful and builds self-esteem. If teachers have the flexibility for other methods, I think that would be very beneficial.

DB: Absolutely. And you have to ask the question, "*What* exactly am I assessing and *why* am I assessing?" For instance, my wife is a teacher, and she had a student who was very stressed at the end of the school year. It was anxiety in general and having many classes where he wasn't doing too well. As the school year was ending, he owed her an essay where he was supposed to argue something. She knew he was a good writer because after a year together, she had seen lots of writing samples. Currently, he was not able to write that essay because of everything that was happening around his life. Now, she had to ask, what exactly am I assessing? He had not written the essay, but giving him a zero—that says that he doesn't know how to write. It doesn't make sense. She realized that he just didn't have the time to write because he was too stressed to sit down and write the essay. She asked him to come in person and said she would give him the chance to talk about it. It's great.

Somebody else might say it's not fair, that's not what the assignment was. [But my wife] has evidence throughout the year that he knew how to analyze text, and she would get him to do it except through speaking. That removed so much anxiety from this poor kid. He could demonstrate the same level of understanding that he would have with a writing assignment, so I totally agree with you. I just want more educators to be encouraged to do this. But again, the kid's mindset was created by adults. The teacher's mindset was created by the system under which they work; it's not really up to the individual teacher. My wife is lucky that she thinks this way and works at a school where she was able to do this. However, I know for a fact from experience that there are schools where if you did that, as a teacher, you would get in trouble. So, that's why in addition to encouraging teachers to be creative and innovative, they need support from those who are above them as well.

JB: Yes. Well, what you're really also talking about is compassion, kindness, empathy, because no one really knows what a student is going through. If they're a rock star student, and then they start coming to school after being remote and suddenly they look thin and they're not communicating and they're not doing their assignments, maybe there's not enough food on the table. Maybe there's something else going on at home. So as teachers, obviously they have so much on their plate, but if they can be a detective, engage and figure out what's going on, they might help that student.

DB: Yeah, it goes into one of the pillars of mind—social and emotional learning, which is essentially the science of understanding, having self-awareness of your emotions, of who you are, and then learning how to manage those emotions, how to have a social awareness and making good decisions, and building strong relationships, and so on. One way to think about that is really to learn how to view people holistically, as a whole human being.

If you think about them as a whole, as a holistic person, then you think about them within your class, outside the school before they get to class, and after your class, then you realize that [something may happen when they're on their way to school] that might impact their [performance]. For example, [they might have] anxiety over what they might [experience in or] after your class. Maybe in the last few minutes of your class, they aren't as engaged. So yes, be a detective, but you will not always be able to actually get the answer right away. People do the best they know how, especially kids. There aren't many kids out there who are intentionally planning the ways in which they are going to be mean to teachers or be disrespectful. Assume that it comes from something that happened to them, the minute, the hour, the day, the month before the actual interaction. Even if you don't know exactly what happened.

JB: You said something really important, which was if a teacher is allowed to go out of that box, it comes down to a policy change; it's not up to the teacher. But if we're going to integrate mental health and wellness, we have to also think differently in giving teachers leeway to be more creative.

DB: Absolutely. There are a few steps that needs to be followed. We need to have a change in policy, but then you need to follow with training and support. Because what I've also observed is that sometimes there can be a policy that says you should care about kids' mental health. Well, that's a good first step. But how do you do that? What exactly does that mean? So, provide resources to help change the policy. But then don't be afraid to look into something new. Change the way we train teachers. In fact, I believe that teachers' academies or Master of Education, that's where you start, but anybody who goes to school to become a teacher, even at that level, the higher education, they should also change their policies and their programs so that those teachers come out of school having learned these tools already. There are so many things that need to happen, but it definitely includes to teach the individual teacher, teachers in general as a whole in the profession, how we prepare teachers, school leaders and administrators, policies, and so on.

I think those are interactions I've had with adults where a teacher may tell me about a specific student who is not motivated. Well, it's interesting because if you are a science teacher or a math teacher or an English teacher, it may appear that they don't have any motivation in a particular task in your class. But this is the same kid who, when their video game is broken, and they want to play with their friends, they will get on YouTube, watch hours of tutorials, fix their own X Box. So, I'm struggling to understand how this is the same person who is not motivated. It's just not true. It's that we need to learn how to tap into that motivation. I love the model that you shared. There is one more that I've adopted over the past maybe seven years—thinking about ABCs: A for autonomy, B for belonging, and then C for competency or competence. If you want to tap into somebody's intrinsic motivation, create an environment where yes, you are the educator in charge, but create a sense of autonomy.

Like we talked about the student who might want to sing a song to express what they learned, as opposed to write an essay, a sense of autonomy—give them options that they can choose to belong. Make them feel as if they are part of the community. The classroom, just like a football team or soccer team, is a community where they have inside jokes, they have a common language that they understand. And then of course, we need to be competent, right? Just because you have autonomy, and you feel belongingness, and it's smart, but you don't have any competence in math, then that's not going to work out. So those three things together are important, but it seems to me, education tends to focus on only being competent in the subject and doesn't spend as much time overall on belonging and autonomy.

JB: Anything else you'd like to share before we wrap up?

DB: I just want to say that everybody's going through it. Nobody is okay. The teachers are not okay. Your school leaders are not okay. Nobody is. Every single individual is going through it. Forget about your title—if you're a teacher a superintendent, you are going through it. The system has to change, and I am hoping that more and more individuals, since individuals make the system, can look into the past couple of years and not start to go back to normal, if normal is pre-pandemic, but take those lessons that we've learned and move forward with that mindset that emotional intelligence is extremely important. Mental health, wellness, well-being—those are things that you can focus on. Not only are we going to have healthier human beings, but you're going to have higher achievers. Some of the things you care about will also be taken care of if we start with mental health.

In the next chapter, you will learn why becoming a better human should be the topic of conversations and initiatives in a time of tremendous suffering. Creating change within yourself can become a catalyst in igniting others to follow your lead. I hope you will be inspired to raise awareness into why mental health must take precedent right now for the sake of our nation and future generations.

CHAPTER 7

Better Humans

All social change comes from the passion of individuals.
—*Margaret Mead*

Throughout history, the subject of mental health has not been openly embraced, and people with mental health conditions were shunned and had struggled in silence. There has been tremendous stigma and discomfort around sharing a mental illness or the need for "a mental health day." Just telling someone you are seeing a therapist and admitting you take medication can make you feel ostracized and the subject of conversation.

Society is filled with opinions about what works and what doesn't when it comes to addressing mental health issues. Your mental health is your own personal journey, and what works for you might not work for someone else. The important thing is to be open and get the care you need to take the very best care of you. However, this is easier said than done for millions of people. At the moment, resources and trained professionals are scarce, and the need outweighs the availability.

Let me take a moment to be transparent with you. I noticed my own mental health was suffering the past few years, so I did something I never did before. I started seeing a therapist. Making this decision was life changing, but it was not easy to find a therapist. Even though I have insurance, it took months to get an appointment, and my therapist and I didn't mesh. At the end of my initial appointment, I felt so much better having shared some personal issues, but as we were about to wrap up, he proceeded to tell me, "I won't be around for a while." It felt like an experience in dating when you feel there's a connection, and the other person can't get to the exit fast enough.

When he finally had availability for a phone appointment, and I shared how I have been focusing on my self-care to ease my stress and anxiety, he told me, "Focusing on yourself and self-care is selfish." His response was shocking, but the pièce de résistance was when I finally got another in-person appointment. I was just arriving at his office (a thirty-minute drive), when his assistant called to tell me "Dr. Couldn'tCareLess wasn't going to make it." I pulled over and laughed through tears. I was at a rough point, but as usual, I would just have to figure things out on my own. I was officially done with him, and never heard from him again, so the feeling was mutual.

Now, I am very fortunate to have a wonderful therapist, who has helped me unravel my own emotional backstory and take a hard look at all that I have suppressed. Never would I imagine sharing with my show guests, and with you, for that matter, that I see a therapist. If you're like me, you also needed help during the pandemic. Not surprising. We all have a backstory, and mine just happens to be filled with abuse, trauma, and a brilliant mother who suffered from addiction and mental health issues. I just never opened up to very many people, and my pain and suffering were suffocating and holding me back.

After experiencing the life-changing power of *real* therapy, a weight has been lifted. If me opening up encourages you or someone else to do the same, then maybe we can create a domino effect and end the stigma around mental health. It's 2022. Enough is enough with silencing people and making them not feel heard or comfortable being their authentic selves. If you openly share your mental health struggles, I commend you. You are a role model for change and an example of how there is no time for stigma and silence anymore.

When you feel valued, seen, and heard—this is when you can feel truly transparent and embraced. Therapy has taught me it is possible to heal and thrive at any age, and the people and experiences that hurt us don't deserve the space and time we give them.

We all have a role to play in becoming better humans, and it all begins on an individual level, taking a look at ourselves, our pre-existing mindsets, prejudices, lack of information, apathy, and what role we have in bringing about necessary change. You have a voice in addressing issues around mental health, stigma, and public health. Our societal issues are problematic, deeply rooted, and expansive, and we must create change to positively affect the mental health and well-being of the foundation and future of our world.

The creation of new policies, public health initiatives, extensive training and education around mental health preventative strategies, and educational and business initiatives must become a blueprint for school curriculum, business policies, and in all settings within society. This requires shifting priorities, elevating marginalized voices, making space for ongoing conversations about mental health, and changing the way we treat one another. It's time to take a stance on creating a lasting impact in our own lives and within society. It's time to stop numbing out with technology addiction, ignoring issues right in front of us, and looking the other way when we know there is something wrong with the status quo. I hope you will be inspired to take action on the following ways you can become a better human and inspire change throughout interconnected frameworks of society.

The following sections provide an overview of key areas that impact the mental health of humans and what can be done to create sustainable, much needed change for the betterment of our nation, and the world.

BETTER HUMANS: Let's Start with YOU

Born This Way vs. Changeable—there are four factors that affect your mental health.

As you check out the following diagram, think about whether these determinents of health are within or not within your control.

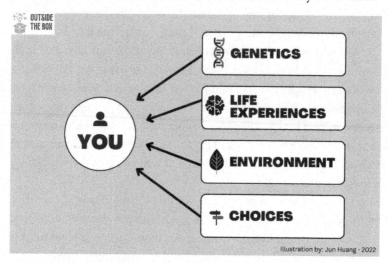

Illustration by: Jun Huang - 2022

Your mental health is affected by genetics, life experiences, environmental issues, and the choices you make. Let's unpack each one.

Genetics

You can't change your DNA, but you can be a detective and figure out your backstory. Don't set limits on yourself because you find out there is something concerning in your family history. Do your homework and bring awareness to your own life. You will be better equipped to create a life of personal strategies that work for you by knowing *why* and *who* you are, but you are not a label or a diagnosis.

For example, I have ADHD. Funny enough, I didn't realize until writing this book, and then it became very clear, and I had a lot of "Aha!" moments. The signs were there, but I just fought through my struggles, which included having a hard time focusing (all my life), anxiety, and depression. I just never paid attention to the signs. Now that I know, I just keep seeing so many TikTok videos about adults having ADHD, and truthfully, I look at it as my creative superpower. I look back to my childhood and see that all of my creative outlets were a testament to my mind on overdrive; they were part of my resilience toolkit and I wouldn't change a thing.

When it comes to genetics, explore your:

- Family history of mental health issues such as depression, anxiety, ADHD, bipolar, disorder, and more
- Immune system issues
- Allergies and food issues
- Physical health conditions

By knowing more about your biological characteristics, you will be better able to make good choices about taking care of yourself long-term, from the food you eat to the routines that help you function at your very best.

Life Experiences

Your mental health can be affected by physical, mental, or emotional distress due to tragedy, crisis, abuse, neglect, and loss. Injury, social isolation and loneliness, discrimination of all kinds, and hardship also impact your mental and emotional health. If you feel that any of these experiences resonate with your own backstory or know someone who is struggling, please reach out to a mental health professional. You can also refer to the resources I have included in the Appendix section.

Environment

In addition to genetics and life experiences, your environment plays a big role in impacting your mental health. Examples of environmental factors include:

- Societal issues such as violence and discrimination of all kinds
- Poverty

- Lack of (nutritious) food or safe drinking water
- Unsafe neighborhoods
- Community or lack thereof
- Exposure to toxic environmental stress resulting in health issues
- Discrimination based on your age, gender, racial, cultural, or ethnic background
- Lack of healthcare and mental healthcare resources, professionals, and treatment
- No options for support that make you feel seen and heard (e.g., a BIPOC therapist, a peer-to-peer support system)
- Stress

Choices

Your lifestyle affects your thoughts and behaviors, as well your health. Everything you do is impacted by your choices, from how you function day-to-day to how you handle stress and the unexpected.

How you treat yourself affects every aspect of your life, from your health and well-being to your relationships. The most important relationship you will have in life is with yourself, and there are numerous decisions you make daily that affect your thoughts and behaviors negatively or positively. Choices that impact your wellbeing include: your words and actions, how you speak to yourself (negatively or positively), your routines and habits (exercise, sleep, and nutrition), your boundaries (saying no, making time for yourself), and your tech consumption (social media, phone use, etc.).

In life, s^&* happens—all the time. Some things happen that are within your control and other times life's circumstances are not within your control (e.g., a global pandemic). Your world is rocked either way, and how you react to life's unexpected moments is a test to your strength and resilience, whether you can handle ambiguity or whether you curl up in a ball and hide away somewhere. The truth is, sometimes we all need to be reclusive because life can be overwhelming and emotionally exhausting, to say the least. Just know when it's time to come back out and be with humans again. Even if you take baby steps, ease back into your life or create a new one. And for any of you who need to hear this—there is no time frame for grief; it's a personal journey. Many of us never get over losing someone. We just move forward to the best of our ability and learn to be patient and kind to ourselves. Just do *you* and take care of yourself. This is all you can do, really.

I am an introvert who dabbles as an extrovert, but I have to run home and recharge my battery. I have always been this way, and this is how I function in life. I go deep inside myself when my world is rocked by loss, for example, and then I start processing my feelings and emotions and figure out a way to build myself back up because I crumbled into a lot of pieces. Oftentimes, I put myself back together and have a completely different outlook and feel thankful for hitting rock bottom and rearranging my perceptions and feelings.

Prior to 2020, the U.S. was already facing public health challenges, and then COVID-19 created unprecedented chaos exacerbating pre-existing issues: the opioid crisis, rates of depression, anxiety, suicide, self-harm, loneliness social isolation, homelessness, and disparities such as access to healthcare, treatment for mental health issues, food insecurity, and increasing ongoing violence and trauma. Anyone working in public health or education felt the enormous toll of the pandemic. If you took a moment to pause, I am sure you felt the ripple effect of a global virus in your own world.

You are about to dive into the How to Become a BETTER HUMAN illustration, which highlights how becoming a better human begins with you—your thoughts, behaviors, pre-existing mindsets, and willingness to change. As you learned from many of the conversations in this book, you are an integral part of the equation for change, but the bigger impact is determined by policies, mental healthcare, schools, businesses, society, and evaluating new initiatives to determine their effectiveness. We cannot assume that sparkling new initiatives and campaigns work if we don't talk to the end users and see their long-term impact. To improve the mental health and well-being of our hurting nation, you and I can become catalysts for change; this starts by learning more about mental health conditions, creating mental fitness mindsets, and spreading knowledge and skills about what to do when you or someone you know needs help.

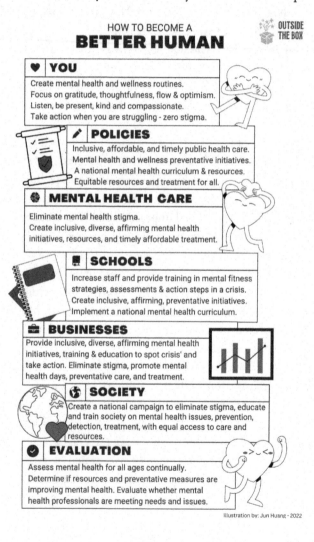

HOW TO BECOME A
BETTER HUMAN
OUTSIDE THE BOX

♥ YOU
Create mental health and wellness routines.
Focus on gratitude, thoughtfulness, flow & optimism.
Listen, be present, kind and compassionate.
Take action when you are struggling - zero stigma.

✎ POLICIES
Inclusive, affordable, and timely public health care.
Mental health and wellness preventative initiatives.
A national mental health curriculum & resources.
Equitable resources and treatment for all.

❀ MENTAL HEALTH CARE
Eliminate mental health stigma.
Create inclusive, diverse, affirming mental health
initiatives, resources, and timely affordable treatment.

▤ SCHOOLS
Increase staff and provide training in mental fitness
strategies, assessments & action steps in a crisis.
Create inclusive, affirming, preventative initiatives.
Implement a national mental health curriculum.

💼 BUSINESSES
Provide inclusive, diverse, affirming mental health
initiatives, training & education to spot crisis' and
take action. Eliminate stigma, promote mental
health days, preventative care, and treatment.

✪ SOCIETY
Create a national campaign to eliminate stigma, educate
and train society on mental health issues, prevention,
detection, treatment, with equal access to care and
resources.

✔ EVALUATION
Assess mental health for all ages continually.
Determine if resources and preventative measures are
improving mental health. Evaluate whether mental
health professionals are meeting needs and issues.

Illustration by: Jun Huang - 2022

BETTER HUMANS: YOU first!

Creating mental health and wellness routines are preventative measures that help you manage stress, anxiety, and the unexpected curveballs of life. Mental fitness is just as important as other essential routines, such as brushing and flossing your teeth, but even more so. Mental fitness is your foundation for life and remains constant. Exercise, eating well, sleep routines, tech disconnect, and connecting with people, places, and experiences are all part of your mental, physical, emotional, and spiritual health. The lure of technology can affect every part of your body and your interpersonal relationships. Know when to unplug and focus on your real life.

Are you easily bored? Switch up your routines from time to time. Trying new activities and learning new things can be a great habit for life. Your preventative care can adapt to suit your needs and interests and where you are in your life. As long you focus on prioritizing your mental, physical, and emotional fitness, you will see the benefits with whatever you choose to do.

Many of you often hear: "If you are struggling, seek professional help." Great advice, but easier said than done. You might not have a healthcare plan that covers the cost of a therapist. You might be standing in a long line at school to see your school psychologist or waiting to hear back from your healthcare provider and never receive an appointment to meet with a therapist. You also might not feel comfortable talking about what is bothering you with anyone who does not reflect or relate to who you are as a person, such as your race, culture, gender identity, and ethnicity.

If you are student who is struggling or see someone else struggling, reach out to your teachers, staff members, administration, parents, campus counseling office, mentor, or campus wellness organization. If you are an adult, reach out to your healthcare provider and see what your options are for care or connect with a peer and see if they have a resource or organization that would be well suited to you. I have provided a list of organizations in the Resources chapter. Whatever you choose to do, please do something. Silence will not make your pain, or someone else's pain, go away. There are people who care and are ready to listen and help. You are not alone in your journey, so please reach out.

* * *

Back in 2019, when my first book came out entitled, *Get the Funk Out! %^&* Happens, What to Do Next!* I began giving talks about resilience, self-care, and lifelong habits for mental health and well-being. In March 2020, I began sharing my method of resilience that has now become a framework for numerous virtual and in-person talks with students and adults; it is called the GTFO Method and includes four essential mindfulness experiences to focus on: Gratitude, Thoughtfulness for yourself and others, Flow, and Optimism. As you learn to integrate this method into your life, this framework will contribute to the foundation of becoming a better human.

Gratitude

Focus on someone or something you are grateful for; this mindfulness experience has numerous benefits:

- Makes you thankful
- Increases your appreciation
- Acknowledges the goodness in your life
- Makes you feel good, builds strong relationships
- Promotes empathy and compassion

Write down your feelings in a journal about why you are grateful for someone or something. You could take this a step further and write a letter or make a phone call to the person you are grateful for. Let them know how you feel about them. The power of hearing someone's voice is a lot more meaningful than a text or email.

Thoughtfulness—for YOU!

"I like to focus on my relationship with myself by listening to what my needs are and reminding myself that I can meet them. If I'm feeling frazzled, I like to remind myself that I am there for me by choosing to focus on something calming like a single player video game." —Rocket Garcia

"I listen to music while out on a walk and sing. I watch cathartic shows and movies and create art to get out of my head." —Kara Worrells

Focus on you, first. When you are good to you, you can be good to the people in your life. Tuning in to your needs, desires, and aspirations can be hard to do, especially when you are juggling so many roles and responsibilities. However, being thoughtful to yourself is essential throughout your lifetime, and this means setting boundaries, putting yourself first, and saying no to people and experiences when you know you are overly committed or just need a break. Take moments to pause and recharge. Your body will tell you what it needs. You just need to be listening.

Here are some thoughtfulness tips:

- Have compassion for YOU
- Ask yourself "How am I *really* feeling?"
- Talk to someone if you are struggling
- Make self-care a priority
- Create positive habits and routines:
  - Water intake
  - Food choices
  - Gut health—your microbiome
  - Eating behaviors
  - Sleep
  - Healthy relationships
  - Manage stress, anxiety, mental health

- Tech disconnect
- Have downtime—don't be "busy" all the time and constantly in motion
- Make good decisions regarding your mental, physical, emotional and spiritual health
- Practice mindfulness and breathwork
- Be a detective when it comes to your well-being (a toxic person/behavior can be detrimental)
- Tune in to your emotional responses to situations out of your control
- Have physical outlets that boost you mentally and physically

Thoughtfulness—for Others

One of the best ways to boost your mood is to be of service to others. Just tuning in to someone else's needs, being considerate, kind and helpful in any way can be a win-win for both of you.
Ways to be thoughtful include:

- Being compassionate
- Showing empathy
- Being patient
- Doing acts of kindness—offer to help, donate your time, money, resources
- Reaching out by phone or messaging
- Tuning in to someone else's mental, physical and emotional health
- Listening actively
- Offering unconditional support
- No ghosting—being honest and polite when you want to quit someone or something

Flow

The theory of flow was named by Hungarian American psychologist Mihaly Csikszentmihalyi. In the field of positive psychology, flow is the mental state of being in a zone, immersed in something that lifts you up and brings you joy; this activity might be challenging, but it is not impossible. You are focused on learning something new, disconnecting from the monotony of your life, setting boundaries, and making time to connect with new activities and interests. When you get into this "zone," it feels like a mental vacation. The experience boosts your self-esteem, level of happiness, and motivation. Spend time doing something you enjoy and time flies, such as painting, playing an instrument, exercising, writing, and other creative pursuits.

Optimism

In May 2020, I took an incredible online psychology course by Dr. Laurie Santos called the Science of Well-Being. Dr. Santos is a Professor of Psychology and Head of Silliman Residential College at Yale University, and she hosts the popular podcast, *The Happiness Lab*. At the beginning of the pandemic, I took her Science of Well-Being course, and the timing was perfect. I was feeling anxious and overwhelmed by the pandemic. When I started her course, I felt such a shift in my mood and outlook. I began to be more mindful and present with my life experiences.

Here are some tips to boost optimism in your life:

- Focus on the quality of your relationships—spend time with people who are good for you and support you
- Seek meaning and purpose
- Do things that create positive change within you and society
- Participate in activities that are out of your comfort zone but are good for your personal growth, connecting you to new people and experiences and your community

- Try new things, whether it's a new place you never visited before or a new type of food or weekend experience. Having a growth mindset is a great way to boost your mood and experience life to its fullest.
- Become a life-long learner creating a non-linear life

Know that the "Keys to Success" have changed and you just need to learn how to handle loss, rejection, and disappointment in life, because how you bounce back through the ups and downs matters most of all.

BETTER HUMANS: POLICIES

Policymakers must realize the urgency in addressing the mental and emotional health of students and adults *now*. For example, the poor academic performance of students as highlighted in the media should be no surprise. Not all students did well academically or emotionally in the pandemic, and additional factors such as income level, lack of mental health support, tremendous loss, having a disability, or being discriminated against or marginalized also play a role in mental and emotional health. Stress, depression, anxiety, and low test scores are to be expected. With limited or no mental health and wellness resources and staff, students need the tools and skilled personnel that reflect students' diverse, cultural, and racial backgrounds.

Mental health legislation is not enacted as swiftly as it should be. If mental health bills had taken precedent early on into the pandemic, perhaps this would have eased some of the mental health conditions brought on by COVID-19, affecting individuals and families. The inability of our mental healthcare system to handle the individual and societal effects of the virus has been evident in the daily news and data regarding mental health struggles. Below are some recent bills making headlines, and a look at the road to making them a reality (or not) in the mental health pandemic.

Policy:	Senate Bills 14 and 224 - two Mental Health Education bills
Author:	Senator Anthony J. Portantino's (D-CA)
Summary:	Signed into law to implement mental health training and education in schools to increase awareness about mental health issues, end stigma, and encourage students to speak up when they are struggling
Status:	October 2021 - California Governor Gavin Newsom signed State Senator Anthony J. Portantino's (D-CA) two Mental Health Education bills
The Reality:	This new initiative is supported by the National Alliance on Mental Illness (NAMI) of California, California Alliance of Child & Family Services, California Youth Empowerment Network, and other mental health organizations, including mental health advocates. Other states need similar mental health legislation. This policy is great for California, but these new laws cannot be implemented fast enough. With SB 224 enacted, this law requires that the California Department of Education create a plan to integrate mental health programs into public school instruction by January 1, 2024. Hopefully, teachers and students do not have to wait until 2024 because this seems like a great new initiative that could benefit students and teachers as soon as possible. Imagine how many lives could be affected by the right mental health instruction and prioritization of mental health needs.

Policy:	Mental Health Matters Act (H.R. 7780)
Author:	Mark DeSaulnier (D-CA)
Summary:	September 22nd, 2022 - the House of Representatives passed the Mental Health Matters Act (H.R. 7780). According to Mychael Schnell, Congressional Reporter at The Hill, this legislation would address the needs of students, families, and educators who have suffered tremendously in the pandemic.

Status:	Nothing is happening yet because even though the House passed this impactful mental health legislation (and it made headlines), it is up to the Senate to decide next, and then off it goes to the President, who has the final say. H.R.7780 is filled with great intentions, but what's taking so long? Unless no one clearly sees the urgency on this.
The Reality:	I can't imagine members of the House and Senate do not have some personal experience with mental health struggles (a child, grandchild, or a friend who is struggling). Something this important could change the trajectory of people's lives, but it is not approved yet. Schnell, Congressional Reporter at The Hill, says that if the legislation is passed by the Senate and becomes a law, then grants could fund school-based mental health services and increase the number of mental health professionals in schools that are struggling to provide mental health services. Let's hope this bill is passed by the Senate and signed into law sooner rather than never.

Next up…I was so happy to read about this next potential mental health bill.

Policy:	Mental Health Justice Act
Author:	Katie Porter (D-CA)
Summary:	In 2021, the Mental Health Justice Act was introduced by representative Katie Porter (D-CA). According to Congress.gov, this bill would provide grants "for states and local governments to train and dispatch mental health professionals to respond, instead of law enforcement officers, to emergencies that involve people with behavioral health needs." The Substance Abuse and Mental Health Services Administration (SAMHSA) would oversee the program with the Department of Justice (DOJ). "SAMHSA may cancel grants that increase incarceration or institutionalization. Grantees must use funds for purposes including de-escalation and anti-racism training. The Department of Health and Human Services and the DOJ must evaluate this program."
Status:	The Mental Health Justice Act was *introduced* in 2021.

The Reality:	...and not much else happened.

Policy:	The Restoring Hope for Mental Health and Well-Being Act of 2022 (H.R. 7666)
Author:	Frank Pallone, Jr. (D-NJ)
Summary:	According to Congress.gov, this bill "expands, and modifies programs, grants, and activities that focus on mental and behavioral health." If this becomes a law, numerous initiatives will address mental and emotional health issues, substance abuse, suicide prevention, behavioral health (e.g., eating disorders), mental health services in schools, crisis response, and more.
Status:	There *is* hope for all of you who are struggling, but as of June 2022, this bill has only just passed the House.
The Reality:	I would really like to see this become law sooner rather than later. Representative Pallone has really touched on a lot of important issues with this bill.

Policy:	S. 2661—the National Suicide Hotline Designation Act of 2020
Author:	Senator Cory Gardner (R-CO)
Summary:	October 2019, Senator Cory Gardner (R-CO) introduced a bill that would require the FCC to authorize 988 as a new national hotline for suicide prevention and mental health crisis.
Status:	In 2020, this bill became a law.
The Reality:	Now, if only other mental health legislation would pass this quickly...

In March 2022, the U.S. Department of Health and Human Services (HHS.gov) announced that the Biden-Harris Administration's HHS Secretary Xavier Becerra would be starting a new initiative called "the National Tour to Strengthen Mental Health" as a way to address the mental and behavioral health crisis compounded by the

COVID-19 pandemic. With planned visits around the United States, Secretary Becerra assessed mental health challenges such as substance abuse, suicide, and other mental health conditions. Their goal is to "engage with local leaders to strengthen the mental health and crisis care system in our communities." Secretary Becerra and members of the HHS are supporting the Biden-Harris Administration's strategy "to transform mental health services for all Americans."

To learn more about the status of current mental health legislation, visit: www.congress.gov.

What's Needed (the bare minimum)

Legislation around mental health and well-being needs to move along much faster through the bureaucratic process. Time is of the essence, and our nation is clearly struggling. Public policies can potentially have a positive impact on people who struggle with mental health conditions and families, as well as marginalized, incarcerated, low-income communities. With timely changes in health policies, people can receive the services and treatment they need, which can in turn have a positive impact on improving their mental and emotional well-being in the long-term. Those who are struggling need to know that there are people who care, who want to help, and that there are solutions underway to make their life easier and more manageable.

Here are some policy suggestions:

- Inclusive, affordable, and timely public healthcare
- Mental health and wellness preventative initiatives
- A national mental health curriculum and resources for schools and businesses that reflects diversity, equity, and inclusion
- Equitable care and treatment for all individuals
- Integration of mental health initiatives and assessments in schools, businesses, and society

- Public health programs that raise awareness on physical, mental, emotional health, affordable insurance and access, mental healthcare and treatment, among others

In 2021, the U.S. Surgeon General Vivek Murthy, M.D., testified that there needs to be an increase in the mental health workforce due to the nation's tremendous youth mental health crisis. His advisory entitled, "Protecting Youth Mental Health," emphasized the urgency in addressing the mental health of youth and families and pre-existing mental health issues prior to the pandemic. Surgeon General Murthy outlined steps that "individuals, families, community organizations, technology companies, governments, and others can take to improve the mental health of children, adolescents, and young adults." He shared that our future depends on how we help today's youth through this mental health crisis.

Unfortunately, thousands of mental healthcare providers left their profession and were not able to meet the unprecedented need for mental health services. In his report, he points out that the disruption caused by COVID-19, from remote learning to missed milestones, inequities in access to healthcare, food, and housing, has affected vulnerable youth who were already struggling in marginalized communities. Surgeon General Murthy shared that these youth are homeless, disabled, LGBTQ, low-income, living in rural areas, living with immigrant parents, and part of the child welfare or juvenile justice system. He also noted that more research is needed to look at the impact of technology on youth mental health.

As of September 2022, the American Academy of Pediatrics (AAP) was awarded $10 million from the U.S. Department of Health and Human Services (HHS), through the Substance Abuse and Mental Health Services Administration (SAMHSA), and will create the *Center of Excellence: Creating a Healthy Digital Ecosystem for Children and Youth.*

MENTAL HEALTHCARE

The pandemic elevated stress and burnout, exacerbated pre-existing mental health conditions, increased disparities, and increased the need for treatment nationally. From schools to businesses, mental healthcare must be inclusive, affirming, and timely.

What's Needed

- National initiatives to eliminate mental health stigma
- Conduct needs assessments in schools and businesses to determine the extent of mental health conditions and struggles and create solutions based on needs
- Provide training and education for students and adults to spot a crisis and take action
- Develop inclusive, diverse, and affirming mental health initiatives and curriculum
- Create preventive peer-to-peer mental fitness initiatives and promote mental health days
- Provide well-trained mental health professionals, resources, and timely affordable care
- Support and compensate mental health professionals for the essential work they do
- Invite experienced mental health speakers who share lived experiences about their mental health conditions, coping strategies, intergenerational trauma, insights into mental health dialogue, and ways to eliminate stigma
- Promote cultural, spiritual, and creative arts practices that promote mental health and well-being
- Support grassroots organizations that promote diverse, equitable, and inclusive mental health and wellness programs for all ages

In President Biden's first State of the Union address, he presented a large-scale strategy to address our nation's mental health pandemic.

The U.S. Health and Human Services Secretary Xavier Becerra has made the President's comprehensive plan a top priority at HHS. Since January 2021, the Biden-Harris Administration has made unprecedented investments to support the promotion and launching of the 988 Suicide and Crisis Hotline, investing $432 million to handle the crisis center's ability to handle the magnitude of calls in our current mental health pandemic.

Some of the key components in Biden's plan include promoting the mental health of frontline workers to alleviate burnout, crisis response and suicide prevention, substance abuse and the mental health of veterans, a National Caregiving Strategy to support family caregivers, and numerous other initiatives.[9]

After President Biden discussed the magnitude of the mental health crisis in his State of the Union address, MTV Entertainment Group launched the first Mental Health Youth Action Forum in collaboration with the Biden-Harris Administration, featuring eighteen leading mental health non-profits. In May 2022, thirty young mental health activists and creators presented ideas to representatives from government, nonprofit, and media and technology companies, as a way to inspire creative digital messaging around mental health and impact today's struggling youth. MTV recognized the influential, creative power of these young activists to turn mental health awareness into action; this event included panels and presentations around mental health, personal journeys, and inspiring initiatives to reach at-risk communities.

The pandemic caused a huge spike in demand for mental healthcare, outweighing the availability of providers in all contexts of society (e.g., hospitals, schools, insurance companies). Many

---

[9] You can read more about the White House multi-level strategy here: The White House, "FACT SHEET: Biden-Harris Administration Highlights Strategy to Address the National Mental Health Crisis," May 31, 2022, https://www.whitehouse.gov/briefing-room/statements-releases/2022/05/31/fact-sheet-biden-harris-administration-highlights-strategy-to-address-the-national-mental-health-crisis/.

therapists stopped taking on new patients or have left the profession. Where does that leave people of all ages and backgrounds who desperately need help? Alone and severely struggling. Amy Kennedy of The Kennedy Forum points out that the list of healthcare providers parents receive from healthcare plans leaves them with little to no options. When parents call the counselors, therapists, and other mental health professionals on these lists, they are told they are not accepting new clients, their insurance is not accepted, or they are no longer in business or out of their coverage area. Parents feel helpless with no assistance and in financial disarray if they choose to pay out of pocket out of necessity. To see your child suffering and you have no way of providing a solution leaves you feeling helpless, to say the least.

Emergency rooms experienced a huge influx of youth seeking help. Unfortunately, our mental healthcare system was not set up to handle the demands of this mental health pandemic. With a shortage of counselors, social workers, psychologists, and much needed resources, the U.S. is struggling and continues to face an uphill battle no one was prepared for. As comedian, commentator, and television host John Oliver points out in his video about our mental healthcare system, "If you're looking for a provider of color, you may have real trouble as white people make up 84% of U.S. psychologists meaning that some patients may have a much harder time finding someone they can relate to." In certain parts of the country, especially rural areas, the demand for care is even greater, and needs go unmet.

Could this explain the emotional, behavioral, and psychological problems that are rampant and the daily incidents of violence among adolescents and young adults? When I hear that a fifteen-year-old was responsible for a deadly shooting, I have to wonder what his story is, whether anyone saw any red flags prior to this horrific incident, whether he was abused, and if he was in treatment or his parents could not afford help. What will it take to stop our epidemic of violence and horrific deaths? I wish I could answer that question.

I am not going to give you some rosy outlook for the future that is filled with idealism and tell you that upping your dose of self-care will make all these anxious feelings go away. All I know is, every day I am more worried and anxious, and by the time this book is finished, there will be even more violent incidents of violence shaking you and I to the core.

I hurt for people who suffer, who experience loss, senseless deaths, and injustice. Having lost my father to cancer in 2015, I am relieved to know he is not here to live in our world at the moment. Some days are just too much. I push through the news like everyone else and look for the glimmer of hope and ways to connect with myself and others, who have no idea how heavy I feel some days. When I read stories like Aiden Hofer Phelan-Ruden's (see next section), with a life lived in so much pain and suffering, I see so many lessons learned. In 2010, when my friend died by suicide, there was so much to learn from her passing; it took me awhile to dig deep, but the lessons were invaluable and painful. I didn't know Aiden, but in the context of this book, you should know his name, because I want his passing to be a catalyst for change in individuals, schools, policies, and our mental healthcare system.

SCHOOLS

Where we are: Nationally, there are not enough resources in schools, a lack of training and education around mental health conditions and action steps to take, insufficient number of mental health professionals to meet the expansive needs, and a need for preventive programs that can improve the mental health of students and adults. With the massive exodus of teachers and mental health professionals, where does that leave students? Let me answer that with a story that is all too common.

Two weeks before I was to submit this book to my publisher, I thought I was done including the people and issues that I wanted to share with you. That was until I read a headline on Yahoo News, "'Does it have to be your kid?' Family calls out mental health system after teen's suicide." Remember the name Aiden Hofer Phelan-Ruden. According to Michaela Ramm, a writer for the *Des Moines Register*, Aiden was described as bright, curious, and a funny kid. He and his brother lived with their grandparents because their parents had substance abuse issues. Aiden was repeatedly bullied in school, harassed online, and beaten up. When his grandfather passed away, he was devastated.

Aiden remained close to his grandmother, and he was seeing a therapist. However, she felt he needed an in-patient treatment center, but the wait was over six months long. Within that time frame, Aiden died by suicide. Ramm points out that Iowa's mental healthcare system, like many areas, is underfunded, understaffed, and lacking critical resources to address the needs of children who struggle with mental illness.

Aiden Hofer Phelan-Ruden is a reminder that there is a massive problem in public healthcare and the mental healthcare system. Millions of children struggle, like Aiden, with mental health issues and never receive the care they so desperately need. Policymakers and lawmakers must prioritize the need for mental health resources in all schools, increase the number of trained staff to meet the demand, and provide resources to promote mental fitness and well-being in K–12, colleges, universities, and beyond. The problem is, there aren't enough people to help, and it is unclear whose responsibility it is to provide resources and mental health training and education for schools. Teachers have enough on their plates and cannot be expected to develop a curriculum for mental health.

On October 24, 2022, there was another school shooting. However, this time, the shooter left a note, and what a wake-up call this should be. According to AP Press writers, Michael Phillis and Jim Salter, the school shooting took place at Central Visual and Performing Arts High School in St. Louis. The shooter was nineteen-year-old Orlando Harris. He killed a teacher and a fifteen-year-old girl and was armed with an AR-15-style rifle. According to Police Commissioner Michael Sack, Harris had over six hundred rounds of ammunition. He told everyone at the school they were going to die. Police Commissioner Sack read the note, which indicated Harris had no friends, no family, and no relationships. He was socially isolated. Sack referred to this as a "perfect storm for a mass shooter." He urged people to take action when they see someone struggling with mental illness. I believe this is one of the foundational problems we are having in this country. Seeing someone post about violent acts, the guns they own, and exhibiting any other kind of questionable behavior should be a red flag for everyone to report potential warning signs. There needs to be training and education around how to spot potentially harmful behaviors, what to do, how to act, and so on. In this recent shooting, Harris had graduated the previous year, and once again, I wonder if people had seen concerning behaviors. Without proper training and education, how would anyone know what to do or what a potential red flag would be?

What's next: Now is the time to create an inclusive, equitable, and diverse mental health and wellness curriculum in schools across the country that has consistent messaging. You are probably thinking, "What a massive undertaking!" Why, yes, it is! But as I mentioned numerous times, STEM and STEAM were mandated as a priority, so it is time to focus on the foundational requirement of being a healthy human, and that is mental health and well-being. Eliminate mental health stigma. Increase the number of trained therapists and counselors to meet the demand, compensate them, and value their expertise. Provide resources and training to prevent a crisis, spot a crisis, and treat mental health issues and illnesses for all ages. Integrate guest speakers, mental health organizations, and grassroots organizations that reflect diversity, equity, and inclusion so students feel they are represented and heard.

Government funding appears to be available for school mental health programming, but the bigger issue is there needs to be a well-designed, national initiative to create a mental health curriculum for all schools and vary it based on age, demographic, diversity, and inclusivity. The pandemic was a long overdue wake-up call that illuminated the fact there must be mental health programming embedded into K–12 and college curriculums for everyone. Mental health cannot be a one-day topic or a flashy workshop. Mental health practices for teachers, administrators, and students must be embedded throughout each day of the school year.

BUSINESSES

Where we are: If you didn't have to shutter your business in the pandemic, consider yourself one of the lucky ones, and a rarity. Maybe your employees worked remotely and some still do, or they are hybrid or back in-person. You probably faced a lot of personal and professional hurdles, but this was also an opportunity for you to rethink the way you treat your employees and prioritize mental health. The pandemic was a wake-up call that you and your employees are not okay, and it's perfectly fine to admit it. We are not machines. We are humans, and we feel things and need to process the unexpected filled with pain and trauma. One of the best things you can do as a leader is to be transparent. Share your own struggles and how you are doing. Be authentic and create an environment where your staff feels heard, seen, and that you are providing the tools and resources for them to thrive mentally, physically, and emotionally.

To do this, you need a mental healthcare strategy with diversity, equity, and inclusion as a top priority. Bring in speakers and create initiatives where people feel supported, heard, and reflected in your business model. Provide training and education around empathy, compassion, emotional intelligence when managing employees. Numerous articles are out now talking about "The Great Resignation" and "quiet quitting." Focus on ways you can retain your employees and make your work environment a place they look forward to coming to.

Messaging around mental health must be embedded into workplace culture so employees feel they can be their true selves, fully supported and accepted for their identities, culturally, ethnically, racially, and gender affirming. If you are struggling mentally and emotionally, your workplace should provide the resources and support you need to take care of yourself and your family. Need a mental health day? This should be part of the workplace culture.

What's needed: How well do you know your employees, and how are they, *really*? Your business can only be successful if you have staff who are mentally and emotionally fit. This means you need to connect on a human level. Find out if there is something that your employees are personally struggling with, but don't pry. Get to know them one-on-one and show them you are listening and really care. Trauma-informed leadership is a skillset you will need to acquire. If you want your employees to be productive and happy at work (whether they are in person or remote), you need to create a culture that is inclusive, trauma-informed, and compassionate.

Want to connect with your employees and be a leader that people will respect, communicate with, and want to work for? Of course, you do. If your employees feel seen, heard, and respected, they will be more likely to show up each and every day, giving their time and dedication. Create a workplace culture that supports mental, physical, and emotional well-being. Start by getting to know the people who keep your business afloat. Ask them individually and collectively how they are and if there is anything they would like to discuss or what you can do to support them in their work. If they share any personal struggles and concerns, be fully present. Be compassionate and a great listener; this is definitely a time to silence your cell phone.

As you connect one-on-one, get to know who they are outside of work. Do they have hobbies, self-care routines, or passion projects? You can think of these conversations as a way to also instill new strategies into your company culture around self-care, mindfulness, and tech breaks. By meeting the needs of your employees, you build an environment that prioritizes mental fitness, empowerment, and dedication.

Ask for their input on how to make things better in the workplace. What works and what doesn't? What ideas do they have for making improvements and building a workplace culture that promotes tech breaks, physical activity, and mindfulness? Provide an open forum for you and your staff to open up and share. Create an environment that supports flex time, mental health days, and "chill spaces" to take a breather (e.g., tech-free zones, yoga/meditation spaces, and workout areas).

See someone struggling in silence? Reach out. Listen. Provide help and support. Apathy is not an option. Foster open communication about mental health and eliminate stigma. Provide education and resources to support mental health. Acknowledge any recent losses: "I am sorry about your _____." Ask if there is anything you can do to support them. Find out how you can help them through a challenging time. For starters, provide your employees with tools, resources, and counseling support. Promote an inclusive, supportive, affirmative workplace that prioritizes mental, physical, and emotional health above everything else. Bring in speakers that reflect the needs, interests, and diverse, inclusive backgrounds of your workforce. Speakers' messages should resonate with your employees and promote conversations around essential topics. Provide preventive support, such as peer-to-peer initiatives and counselors. Have zero tolerance for toxic behavior and discrimination of any kind.

SOCIETY

Where we are: Check your news feeds. There are daily reports of youth and young adults on up who are experiencing mental health conditions, feeling depressed, anxious, and suicidal. You have probably noticed there are more acts of violence in schools and other settings. The incidents of gun violence have increased tremendously, as have mental health issues among Gen Z on up. How did we get to this disturbing place that feels like a bad movie? After a deadly crime, we usually hear that the assailant had a social media account showing off guns, violent posts, or other questionable behavior, and that he was an outlier in his community. Social media is then littered with posts reflecting anger, grief, and "thoughts and prayers," but it's time the U.S. follow the tightened restrictions of other countries who have successfully reduced violent crime rates.

There must be harsher punishments, restrictions, and actions to deter people from more fatal incidents with gun violence and tighter regulations about who and why someone wants to buy an assault rifle, handgun, or other weapon. Social media companies must also be held accountable, requiring them to monitor their anything goes, wild world of social media. It should not be the case that once a horrible crime is reported, people come forward and share that there were red flag warnings all along on Instagram or TikTok.

What's needed: There needs to be a national campaign on all social media platforms, radio, podcast, TV channels, and advertising platforms to eliminate stigma, educate and train society on mental health issues, prevention, detection, treatment, and provide equal access to resources for everyone. Instead of being quick to form a conclusion when we see a potential situation, an in-person or online training and education program would provide a foundation for making informed decisions about situations that might be a pre-cursor to a life-threatening situation. And yes, it's long overdue to overhaul our country's gun control laws and enforce more punitive punishments, so we can reduce and hopefully eliminate violent acts by teens and young adults who plan to purchase or take their parent's assault rifles out into their community. Other countries have taken the lead in responding promptly to deadly acts of gun violence. After every incident, the U.S. has done nothing to address the epidemic of violence.

In a May 2022 article, *Time Magazine* reporter, Eloise Barry, points out that the U.S. has the highest incidence of gun deaths. One of the most recent and horrific incidents that occurred was in Uvalde,

Texas, leaving nineteen children and two teachers dead by the hands of an eighteen-year-old with an AR-15-style rifle. When gun violence occurred in New Zealand and Norway, immediate actions took place to change their gun laws. The UK received pressure from families of victims and the community; they acted swiftly and banned all handguns, resulting in lower incidents of gun violence. What will it take for the U.S. to do the right thing, and how soon? Our country locked down swiftly and promptly when COVID-19 was ravaging our country in March 2020; there were restrictions that made you and I shelter in place. There weren't months of bureaucratic red tape, endless meetings without planned actions. The U.S. was shuttered for the safety and well-being of our country. So, why isn't gun violence taken as seriously and promptly for the safety and well-being of our country? What a deterrent and game changer it would be to have strict laws on guns and gun violence. Would it be a perfect solution? Of course not, but we must start somewhere.

There must be a Better Humans campaign for kindness, compassion, empathy, connection, and resilience. Mental health curriculum across every setting designed for different learners would increase mental health awareness, eliminate stigma, and promote conversations and actions about preventive mental fitness and treatment options. Policymakers cannot expect teachers to create their own mental health programming on top of the workload they already have. What about *their* mental health? Policymakers must take into account the mental fitness of teachers and how we need to stop their exodus from a profession that is essential to future generations.

We need a societal construct for how we treat one another in our interpersonal lives, in social settings, school, work, and in our daily interactions. It's time to unlearn destructive mindsets and patterns of behavior that don't benefit society and the mental health of our society. Outdated, biased, and discriminatory mindsets keep us stuck in negative judgments and preconceived notions about mental health and how to treat people.

We must build a culture of acceptance, inclusivity, diversity, equity, and accessibility so that we may thrive as a unified society, not be divided by differences and hate-filled rhetoric from people who have a distorted view of what the world should look like. People who foster hate, destruction, and narrow-minded thinking for the benefit of their own egos and power trips are only fertilizing the negative mindsets and behaviors in younger generations; this must stop because it raises a generation of people who are not mentally well, which becomes evident in their thoughts and behaviors, especially the violent crimes in the U.S.

As you go about your day, think about how you treat the people you interact with, whether you are kind and accepting or whether you are judgmental and harsh. Do you take into consideration that the person who seems unfriendly might have lost someone? Do they look angry to you? They might be fearful, and that comes across in a different emotion. Don't be quick to judge anyone because you have no idea what their path looks like, how alone they are in their struggles, and how heavy their load is.

All of Us Have a Role

Raise your voice. Speak up. Speak out against stigma, discrimination, and apathy. Raise awareness and make waves. Take action to promote what it means to be a better human. This is how change happens. If you or someone you know struggles with mental health issues, you are not alone. We all have a breaking point, and if you feel you need professional help, please do not hesitate to get the care you need. If you do not know where to start or lack the resources, reach out to a teacher, mentor, friend, family member or professional. I have provided a list of resources in the back of this book that include twenty-four-hour support. Mental health affects everything you do, and if the pandemic has taught you anything, it is time to prioritize your mental health needs first.

Normalize conversations and language around mental health conditions, eliminate stigma, and provide resources and treatment for all people in all areas and backgrounds. In addition to a universal mental health curriculum in schools, the same messaging needs to be spread throughout all forms of media; this includes television, radio ads, social media ads and messaging, and in all settings. Talking about mental health needs to be no different than talking about how you stay physically active. Mental fitness is no different, and you should feel comfortable sharing what you do to take care of yourself mentally and emotionally.

Educate yourself on public health and mental healthcare issues, interventions, and solutions such as peer support, group support or one-on-one counseling, therapy, and treatment. If you are a school, bring in experienced guest speakers who reflect lived experiences (e.g., mental health conditions) and diverse and inclusive backgrounds and experiences. They can share personal strategies that are outside of the box (not within a stereotypical framework) but that work for them such as spiritual, cultural, or other personalized resilience techniques. Grassroot organizations and other mental health organizations and initiatives can share relatable content with people of all ages and backgrounds, reflecting the lives of marginalized communities and their lived experiences.

EVALUATION

Evaluation is an important part in determining the long-term effectiveness and satisfaction of any initiative. There are three key areas that go into any Better Humans initiative:

- Assess mental health for all ages continually
- Determine if resources and preventative measures are improving mental health
- Identity whether there are enough mental health professionals to address demand

Assessments: Ongoing

Evaluating the mental health and well-being of people of all ages should be embedded in every context of society. For example, before a therapy appointment, you complete a pre-appointment assessment online or on an app so your therapist can get a gauge of how you are psychologically, emotionally, and behaviorally, and whether there are any red flags. Assessments should be part of schools for teachers, staff and students, and businesses of all sizes. Remote, hybrid, and in-person workers should all receive an assessment. You can indicate if you are struggling with something specifically, experiencing a loss, personal hardship, a crisis at home, trauma, abuse, suicidal thoughts, depression, anxiety, and so on. You can also indicate your concern for someone else within your setting.

Assessments should also determine whether the school or business has sufficient and effective resources and preventative initiatives to improve mental health. If it does not, action must be taken immediately because this means those who struggle will continue to struggle.

Across the country, the common sentiment is that there are not enough mental health professionals to meet the demand in numerous settings. Where does this leave people who need therapy, treatment, and care? It leaves them feeling hopeless, alone, and unattended to. Think about how this feels to their family. If our nation really cares about the mental health of our people, there needs to be a solution to stop the exodus of healthcare providers and retain enough qualified mental healthcare professionals to do the work that so desperately needs to be done now—not a few years from now. In a few years, maybe some new bills will be passed by the House, and a year later the Senate, but then nothing could happen. Bills with great ideas are wonderful, but actionable steps are what is needed now. We cannot afford to wait for change that should have happened long ago. There is too much at stake.

CHAPTER 8

Outside The Box

The Power of Purpose-Driven Initiatives for Mental Health

"We will continue to be in a mental health pandemic, unless we completely shift the way that our society is run. And I think that can be said for every single issue that we see today."
—Rocket Garcia, 24

The year 2020 was a tremendous time of reflection for me. In February 2020, I was doing some speaking events and never imagined that the event hosting a panel discussion about the Science of Happiness would be my last in-person event for a very long time. In early March, something in my gut told me to cancel my March 2020 plans to speak at a museum in Westport, Connecticut and postpone a trip to New York City; this same museum would later be mentioned in the media because a party was thrown and COVID-19 was the uninvited guest.

Throughout 2020 and 2021, I received messages from students looking for mentoring and advice as to what to do after their much-anticipated plans were no longer a reality. Having had an incredible mentor at Syracuse University, who randomly took two hours out of his day to meet with me as a confused college sophomore, Dr. Phillip

Doughty exemplified the true meaning of kindness, compassion, and mentoring. We are still friends to this day, and I have always felt that I would do the same for someone else. Little did I know that "someone else" would turn into numerous young adults tremendously impacted by a pandemic.

In response to the mental health pandemic, I launched OUTSIDE THE BOX initially as a podcast in 2020. In addition to the podcast, OUTSIDE THE BOX also includes workshops and events focused on mental health, self-care, social issues, and strategies to promote sustainable, transformative change. During the summer of 2022, I created the OUTSIDE THE BOX Creative Arts Series, led by Gen Z instructors on up. The idea for this virtual program came about because I knew that creativity has the power to inspire and boost positivity. I gathered numerous mental health advocates, wellness educators, and creative content experts, and launched a series of uplifting workshops. Some of the topics included: The Power of Poetry, Illustrative Journaling, Yoga and Meditation, Songwriting, Intro to Hip-Hop, Making Meaning from Adversity, The Power of Doodling for Mental Health, and Using Tech to Advocate and Create. Seeing these instructors share their brilliance in numerous ways was a joy to witness.

Launching OUTSIDE THE BOX was the perfect purpose-driven solution to give my own life a boost, except the beginning was a tad bumpy—like forgetting to hit the record button on my first zoom interview. Once I found my groove, being an online creator gave me a much needed dose of positivity, a great way to connect with hundreds of new faces I might never have met before, and a mission to help others who were riding a wave in turbulent times.

Through this creative process, I recognized that purpose-driven initiatives have the power to transform lives, foster connection in a time of disconnect and boost mental health. They also improve emotional well-being and instill optimism while creating meaning, empathy, and collaboration. When you create meaningful initiatives, you create solutions that promote a kinder, more thoughtful, and compassionate world, and couldn't we use a little more of that right now?

As my series Outside the Box evolved into a podcast and event series, I began to think of ways to create more purpose-driven content; it was important for me to inspire people of all ages to get involved in meaningful and uplifting experiences and to have a mental vacation from their personal struggles. Here's a story of a purpose-driven initiative that I never saw coming.

I created the concept of the CARE Initiative after my 2021 fellowship with the Age Boom Academy: "Combatting Loneliness in Aging: Toward a 21st Century Blueprint for Societal Connectedness." It is a signature program of the Robert N. Butler Columbia Aging Center in partnership with the Columbia Journalism School. The journalism fellowship brought me tremendous insight into ageism, research on mental health, social isolation, depression, and the negative impact of the pandemic on all age groups.

The CARE Initiative began September 2021 when I was asked to donate excess food by a local donut shop while I was trying to get a refund for an order gone wrong. I pulled through the drive-thru with a bag filled with items that needed to be returned. The employee told me twice that the store was closed, and she could not refund me the money. A very kind employee overheard and thanked me for not yelling, because the computers were down that day, and I didn't have a receipt. As a thank you, he offered me donuts. Years earlier, I would have happily accepted, but now I declined. He asked me to pull around the back door because he wanted to show me something. Curious, I agreed. When he opened the back door, there were over four hundred items on a huge rack, and he said they will end up in the trash. Seeing my reaction, he asked, "Would you please consider taking some donuts and feeding people who are experiencing homelessness?" There was only one response.

Over the next few months, I gathered up items every night and dropped food off at seven local organizations that care for people who are experiencing homelessness or families experiencing food insecurity. Another local bagel shop heard about my initiative and joined in with weekly donations that continue to this day.

I launched the CARE Initiative to create meaningful connections and boost positivity during a time of tremendous disconnect and mental health struggles. The initiative fosters meaning and purpose through four core principals.

CARE stands for:

Connection: connecting to one another has never been more essential addressing the issues that are on the forefront and coming up with local initiatives (e.g., homelessness, food insecurity, ageism, sexism, racism, gender equality, environmental issues, etc.)

Attention: mental, physical, emotional, and spiritual health

Resilience: how to remain adaptable and know how to pivot when life throws you curveballs!

Education: addressing the issues that are on the forefront and coming up with local initiatives (e.g., homelessness, food insecurity, ageism, sexism, racism, gender equality, environmental issues, etc.)

The CARE Initiative is designed to foster connection in our disconnected world, highlight the importance of thoughtfulness for yourself and others, resilience, and education on social issues, humanitarian efforts, homelessness, gender identity, sexual equality, and helping marginalized communities. My talks now include the power of the CARE Initiative and how we can all become better humans in the process. We must build a culture of social connection, collaboration, meaning and purpose, inclusivity, acceptance, and resilience. Having empathy, kindness, and compassion connects us in ways that have long-term impacts.

The CARE Initiative helps foster meaning and purpose, while promoting connection, wellness, resilience, and education. All ages learn to CARE: connect, pay attention to mental health and wellness, focus on resilience building skills and educate one another on issues that impact society. Students learn how to launch a student-led CARE Initiative club and create sustainable, transformative change.

Purpose-driven lessons from the Blues Zones and the Japanese concept called Ikigai

The blueprint for the CARE Initiative was inspired by my personal experiences, the soaring rates of depression and hopelessness, and the benefits of finding a meaningful, purpose-driven life. The Japanese concept for finding your purpose in life called *ikigai*; it means reason for being and can be a powerful tool when life feels difficult and draining. Finding something that gets you excited to get you up in the morning and gives you a sense of purpose, meaning, and empowerment can be a life changer; this is the intersection between what you love and what you are good at.

New York Times bestselling author, speaker and National Geographic Fellow Dan Buettner spoke about the power of connectedness, intergenerational relationships, and the world's "Blue Zones" in his 2013 TED Talk. Buettner shared that in Okinawa, elders live longer and connect in meaningful, purposeful ways. Their lifestyles and diet in one of the original blue zones show they have a better quality of life with friends that they have known since childhood. Older generations are valued and thrive as they stay connected to their families instead of isolated, depressed, and put into retirement homes. I often refer to intergenerational connectedness between elders and children as the "grandparent effect," and Buettner calls it the "grandmother effect." These Blue Zones reflect the keys to longevity, and a model for mental and physical health for other communities to replicate.

Buettner notes that in Okinawa, there is a tremendous value in community and treasuring the elders, and people look after one another. *Moai*, a tradition affecting why people live longer in Okinawa, is a social support group of friends since childhood that have each other's backs through the trials and tribulations of life. There is no talk of retirement in Okinawa but instead the term *ikigai*, which is as Buettner says: "The reason for which we wake up in the morning." Having a sense of meaning and purpose keeps people thriving and gives them a reason to keep going. He said that another common theme is longevity; they are staying physically active by gardening and walking. They have downtime, manage stress, and have a sense of purpose. They eat a plant-based diet, drink in moderation, and are conscious about overeating. They prioritize connection, value older generations, have spiritual practices, and have relationships that are good for them and not detrimental.

There are four main characteristics of *ikigai*:

- What you love
- What you are good at
- What the world needs
- What you can be paid to do

When it comes to creating a purposeful life or choosing a job, think about what you are passionate about, what brings you joy and feelings of being complete that don't involve money, and what makes you excited and satisfied. Find your reason for being and allow yourself time to figure out what you want to share with the world and the gifts you bring.

Knowing what we know about the transformative power of having meaning and purpose, connectedness, and being thoughtful to ourselves and to others, there is a lot that can be applied to mental health and thriving.

CHAPTER 9

Conclusion

The late and brilliant comedic actor Robin Williams privately struggled with depression and his own mental health challenges. Many people were shocked when he passed away and his personal struggles were revealed. How many of us have a public persona where people think you are perfectly happy, when in fact, the reality could not be more opposite? Mental health affects how we treat ourselves, our loved ones, our coping mechanisms, thoughts and behaviors, and all of our intertwined relationships. Mental health struggles are not always seen by others but instead kept under lock and key by someone who might have no idea they need help, doesn't know who to turn to, or perhaps feels trapped by their hamster wheel of negative thoughts and behaviors. Your self-esteem, self-awareness, and ability to prioritize your self-care and resilience strategies has never been more essential.

Writing about mental health has given me pause to reflect on my own journey through therapy, the trauma of my childhood, and growing up with a mother who suffered with mental health issues. My father fought tirelessly for custody of me and my brother, whom I am estranged with and won't be discussing, except for this. After extensive therapy of my own, I feel so sorry for the pain and suffering he must have witnessed as a young baby living with parents who had violent tempers and explosive personalities. Extensive therapy and a deep dive into his soul would have addressed a lot of his trauma and much-needed healing. As I said to my mother after she asked me to leave her at sixteen and tried speaking to me by phone, "I don't hate you, but I can't have anything to do with you." I will leave it at that.

I had a lot of unanswered questions about my mother in the few past years, which is funny because growing up, I thought she was like anyone else's mother, and everything was sort of "normal." I was seventeen the last time I saw her, and she was pointing a rifle at me, not with the intent of hurting me but as a form of protection. She thought I was an intruder when I arrived at her house in North Stamford, Connecticut late one morning from high school. I had woken her up, and she greeted me with her two vicious-looking Dobermans, a massive gun, and blue-striped footie pajamas. It was about 11 a.m. on a weekday and thank goodness she grabbed her thick glasses and realized it was just me. This was the moment that I realized how blessed I was to move in with my dad and turn my entire life around. I backed down the stairs slowly and said, "Don't shoot! It's me, and I will come back another time." Of course, I knew that would never happen.

When I became pregnant with my first child, I was terrified. I would bolt up from being sound asleep, startle my husband, and tearfully say that I was very scared to be a mother. I didn't want to become like my mother. He assured me this would not be the case, but I was determined not to be the mother I *had* but the mother I *wanted* to have. With so many unanswered questions about my mother, I reached out to every husband she was married to. You could say it was like an investigative report and a healing journey all in one. I wanted their perspectives on what she was really like.

She married her first husband at nineteen when they were both students at Emerson College; they had an annulment soon after and never had kids. He shared that she had a very scary temper and to get out of her way when it happened. The second husband was my father, and I heard plenty of stories from him, but I needed to talk to other people just to see if they had similar experiences.

I was born in Bridgeport, Connecticut, to two very beautiful, smart, hardworking young people who met on a blind date in Boston. She was a speech therapist (twenty years old), and he was an accountant (twenty-eight), and they would both go on to have very rewarding careers. They separated when I was six months old, and I moved from house to house, living with my mother and barely seeing my father. At one point, she married an eye doctor briefly, and we lived in Woodbury, New York. He seemed very nice, but I barely spent any time with him after moving into his big, beautiful house. My mom told me to go to the basement when he arrived home each night because "he didn't like kids." I recently found out this could not be further from the truth. He adored me and considered me his daughter. Without any stability, my only joy in that house was music. I can still remember feeling emotionally moved by Santana's "Black Magic Woman" and "Something" by the Beatles.

At age eight, I saw my first band perform live on a Sunday morning brunch at Wednesday's, a restaurant and club across the street from my apartment in New York City. I was pulled toward the music and danced alone on the dance floor as people drank champagne and ate their soggy French toast. I set my gaze on the man playing an electric guitar and was hypnotized, watching his every move, and suddenly, I was hooked for a lifetime. Music would be my lifeline.

At the age of ten, my mother bought me my first guitar, but at the age of thirteen, we had a house fire, and I lost everything. However, one day, she handed me some cash and told me to head to New York and get another one. I got on an early morning train, flagged down a cab, and asked to be dropped in the music district. I was barely thirteen but navigated my way to Manny's Music, where I purchased a beautiful Garcia nylon acoustic guitar that I still have to this day. Music has been the glue to hold me together when life feels fragile and uncertain. There were many nights I chose to stay home with my guitar instead of heading out to a party or bar with friends; it was hard for me to fight through my social anxiety unless I was drinking. By my mid-twenties, I started weaning off of my long list of numbing habits.

My father used to say, "I wish your mother was the woman I wanted her to be, and we could have stayed together as a family." My response was simply, "But Dad, she was not capable of being the person you wanted her to be." In 2021, I finally reconnected with my stepfather Joe, my mother's husband number three. I had not seen him in fifty years. You read that right. Fifty years. I needed some clarity visiting some old memories on who my mother was and what it was like being married to her.

At first, he didn't want to talk about her at the risk of sounding mean. I told him this is part of my emotional healing, and our conversations blossomed into a beautiful friendship. For a year, we connected on Zoom, and he shared how he had ALS. He sent me texts filled with pictures of my mother I had never seen before and shared stories capturing each one. I was saddened to hear that he never married again because she ruined him emotionally and financially, and he never wanted to upend his life again; it was all too painful and traumatic. I was his only child, a stepdaughter, and he considered me his *real* daughter. I treasure the time I had with him, his candid memories of my mother, laughing with him at the absurdities and healing from the past. He shared his life adventures, passions, loves, and joys. What a gift I will treasure forever.

On June 15, 2022, I texted Joe—and so thankful I did. However, his response made my heart sink: "Thanks for your note. I am in hospital dying from Lou Gehrig's disease. I can't talk. Getting oxygen. Sorry to leave you. Take care of yourself, enjoy life. Best, Uncle Joe."

I somehow managed to track down where he was by calling over twelve hospitals in his area. His niece answered his phone. "Please tell him I love him, and I am thinking of him," I said. She did, and he passed away a few hours later.

* * *

In reading about childhood trauma, I realized just how much I ignored my own backstory. I would ignore even the simplest health problem until it became a serious one. I had no focus in school, tremendous difficulty learning, reading, and taking tests. I was told I was "a sensitive child," crying a lot and not being able to control myself, often hiding behind the bathroom door staring at myself in the mirror, a weepy mess. I didn't know I was living in trauma, abuse, and all things toxic. I was just in survival mode.

My mother was brilliant in so many ways, and it is tragic that she passed away at the young age of fifty-three, spiraling into a life of prescription medication, alcohol, and mental health struggles. Having traveled to Virgin Gorda, St. Thomas, and other British Virgin Islands in the 1970s and 1980s, it was no surprise she chose to move to Tortola later in life and spend her final days on Peter Island.

I have gone through periods of grief throughout my life, but losing my mother felt different. When asked by my therapist recently, "How were you loved as a child?" I could not hold back my tears. I was not loved in a physical sense, never shown any real affection, but I was fortunate to learn early on how to navigate the streets of New York City, so I could get to where I needed to be and become very self-sufficient and comfortable being alone day after day. I am thankful for the resiliency skills I learned by getting myself to school every day from first through fourth grade, and then commuting other ways when I switched schools a few more times. I now see the source of my fears and anxieties rooted in childhood trauma, being given alcohol at nine and drugs at fourteen, which then turned into addiction of my own. There were dinners in expensive restaurants (The Plaza, The

Carlisle, The Waldorf, and more) and shows galore on Broadway. But I would much rather have had someone I could curl up to and bury myself in her neck the way my daughters do with me. I would love to have held onto her as tight as my daughters do, and study her face, because to this day, I cannot recall the color of her eyes.

What I will always remember is the groundbreaking work she did for people who were struggling with their identity. They were shunned by their families but had a safe haven with my mother at our apartment on East 86th Street in New York City. I saw the most incredible transformations of men who would enter our apartment, and after extensive transformative sessions with my mother, leave as confident and oftentimes statuesque women. They oozed confidence, and my mother had found her groove in the most underground and much-needed profession: helping transgender men and women.

Loving yourself first is your number one priority in your lifetime. You can't expect someone else to take on that role. Sure, people can help you heal and "feel complete," but looking for someone to fix and heal you is not the road to mental health. Take the very best care of you first, so you are glowing with self-love. That might sound "woo woo," but you will know it when you feel it. Discover your passions and interests and nurture them. Have the best, non-linear life you can have, and don't let anyone else pave the way with their expectations and opinions. Find your passions, your purpose, and things that get you up and out in the morning, and share your gifts with the world. Having meaning and purpose in your life while connecting with others will do wonders for your mental health.

For those of you who have struggled in this mental health pandemic, let's spread the urgency for mental healthcare reform, mental healthcare policies (now, not in a few years), societal change, and mental healthcare curriculums that are effective and impactful in schools and businesses. Isn't it about time you and I spoke up about the importance of healing individually and collectively as a nation? I am ready to be a catalyst for change. How about you?

EPILOGUE

It is time to speak truth to power and dismantle the status quo.

It is time to speak truth to power and restructure the mental healthcare system that does not serve people of all socioeconomic backgrounds, genders, cultures, ethnicities, and races, and respect and value those who provide critical care.

It is time to speak truth to power and prioritize mental health in all aspects of society, for individuals, and for public policy affecting people in all settings, in all conversations, and taking precedence in everything we do.

It is time to speak truth to power and create a more inclusive, diverse, equitable, and safer society where there is no stigma around mental health, no gun violence, no climate crisis, and no discomfort in saying, "I need help."

It is time to speak truth to power and really listen to one another, to be present, thoughtful, engaged, and kind while paying attention to the outliers who might be struggling.

It is time to speak truth to power and disconnect from our tethered devices that steal quality time from our relationships, our lives, and cause us to be alone and numb out scrolling.

You have wounds that are years deep. Every action and overreaction affects those around you. You are hurting. The world is hurting. We cannot be silent anymore.

Let us focus on synergy, instead of divisiveness, embracing differences, connectedness instead of isolation.

How will *you* become a better human?

The future depends on you.

APPENDIX

If you are struggling, please know you don't have to suffer in silence. If you do not have a friend or family member you can talk to, consider reaching out to a mentor, counselor, teacher, or someone else you trust. If not, there are numerous other options for you right here.

988 Suicide & Crisis Lifeline

A 24-hour, toll-free, confidential support for people in distress. Prevention and crisis resources for you or your loved ones
Call or text 988 or chat at 988lifeline.org.

American Foundation for Suicide Prevention

Website: https://afsp.org/
Whether you have struggled with suicide yourself or have lost a loved one, know you are not alone. Hear about personal experiences from people in your local community whose lives have been impacted by suicide.

Behavioral Health Treatment Services Locator

https://findtreatment.samhsa.gov/
A confidential and anonymous source of information for persons seeking treatment facilities in the United States or U.S. territories for substance use/addiction and/or mental health problems.

Childhelp Hotline

childhelphotline.org

The Childhelp National Child Abuse Hotline

If you believe that a child is in immediate danger, please contact (800) 422-4453 for help.

CRISIS Text Line

A free and confidential chat with a trained counselor 24/7.

Text ACTION to 741741

Text HOME to 741741 from anywhere in the United States, anytime. Crisis Text Line is here for any crisis. A live, trained Crisis Counselor receives the text and responds, all from our secure online platform. The volunteer Crisis Counselor will help you move from a hot moment to a cool moment.

Disaster Distress Helpline

1-800-985-5990 or text "TalkWithUs" to 66746

A 24/7 hotline that provides immediate crisis counseling for people experiencing emotional distress related to a natural or human-caused disaster.

Help Outside of the US

https://findahelpline.com/

Find A Helpline | Free, confidential support. 24/7. Chat, text, or phone.

NAMI HelpLine

If you or someone you know needs help, contact NAMI HelpLine

Monday to Friday from 10 a.m. to 10 p.m. ET
Call: 1-800-950-NAMI (6264)
Email: helpline@nami.org
Text: 62640
Chat: nami.org/help

NAMI Ending the Silence is an evidence-based program designed for middle and high school students, families, and school staff. It is offered in-person by NAMI affiliates across the country and on-line when in-person is not an option.
Learn more: www.ets.nami.org

Mental Health is Health.us has a list of warning signs to look for when you see someone struggling.
Learn more: https://www.mentalhealthishealth.us/for-friend/.

National Domestic Violence Hotline

Domestic Violence Support | The National Domestic Violence Hotline (thehotline.org)
1 (800) 799 –7233

National Eating Disorders Association

1 (800) 931-2237
The NEDA Helpline provides support, resources, and treatment options for yourself or a loved one who is struggling with an eating disorder. Helpline volunteers are trained to help you find the support and information you need. Please note that the helpline is not a substitute for professional help.

Opioid Treatment Program Directory

Learn more: https://dpt2.samhsa.gov/treatment/
Find treatment programs in your state that treat addiction and dependence on opioids, such as heroin or prescription pain relievers.

SAMHSA's Disaster Distress Helpline

SAMHSA's Disaster Distress Helpline provides 24/7, 365-day crisis counseling and support to people experiencing emotional distress related to natural or human-caused disasters.
Call or Text: 1-800-985-5990
samhsa.gov/find-help/disaster-distress-helpline

SAMHSA (Substance Abuse and Mental Health Services Administration)

1-800-662-HELP (4357)
Visit Find Treatment Locators and Helplines, https://www.samhsa.gov/find-treatment

A free, confidential resource for finding therapists and other mental health professionals. Available 24/7.

The U.S. Substance Abuse and Mental Health Services Administration (SAMHSA) has a free, confidential information service (in English or Spanish), open 24 hours/365 days, for individuals and family members facing mental health or substance use disorders.

The service provides referral to local treatment facilities, support groups, and community-based organizations. You can also visit SAMHSA's online Behavioral Health Treatment Services Locator at https://findtreatment.samhsa.gov/ for assistance is finding treatment facilities for substance abuse/addiction and/or mental health problems.

California Youth Crisis Line

800-843-5200 for ages twelve to twenty-four

Substance Use Treatment Locator

Millions of Americans have a substance use disorder. Help is available, treatment works, and people recover every day. Find a state-licensed treatment facility near you.
findtreatment.gov

Veterans Crisis Line

Reach caring, qualified responders with the Department of Veterans Affairs. Many of them are veterans themselves.
Dial 988 then press 1
Text: 838255
veteranscrisisline.net

Youth Service Bureaus Clinic Services

650-877-8642 ext. 6526 (English Intake) | ext. 6586 (Spanish Intake)

National Institute of Mental Health Information Center

866-615-6464

TeenLine

800-852-8336 (6PM To 10PM PT everyday)

Thursday's National Youth Advocacy

818-831-1234

Trans Lifeline

877-565-8860

A peer support phone service run by trans people for the trans community, that operates from 10 a.m. to 5 a.m. EST.

Trevor Lifeline

1-866-488-7386 or text "START" to 678-678

A safe, judgement free support service for LGBTQ and questioning youth who are struggling or thinking about suicide. Available 24/7.

ACKNOWLEDGMENTS

Better Humans is dedicated to you, Generation Z on up, because you have been struggling in the past few years, and perhaps your entire lifetime. You have not always been seen, listened to, or recognized for your strengths and struggles, and the pandemic only made life more challenging. I hope you find inspiration in reading *Better Humans* because you have great power to create sustainable change the world needs desperately right now and in the future.

A huge thank you to my contributors who opened their hearts and shared their insights and invaluable research, personal stories, and wisdom. Our conversations stayed with me long after we were finished. In a time of tremendous disconnect and social isolation, I was humbled and honored to listen to your journeys and learn how we can move forward to become better humans.

Thank you to Erin Raftery Ryan, Executive Director, NAMI Westside Los Angeles, for cheering me on and writing such a heartfelt, creative foreword for my readers. To Consulting Editor, Post Hill Press, Debra Englander, your support, and encouragement in bringing this book to life has meant the world to me. Thank you to my outstanding editors Aleah Taboclaon and Emma Venker, and to my amazing book cover designer, Tiffani Shea. Shoutout to my family for your encouragement and love and giving me space to be me. And to Lenore, who guided me gently through my own backstory and made me feel safe peeling back my protective layers. I am forever grateful.

I learned a lot about my own mental health during this journey, and the mental health of the nation. If I can be a catalyst in helping end the stigma around mental health and encourage the creation of purpose-driven mental health initiatives, then we will finally begin to heal our country. The mental health pandemic is vast, and the future depends on all of us moving forward with compassion, kindness, and the urgency to become better humans.

ABOUT THE AUTHOR

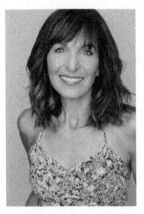

Photo by Joanna Degeneres Photography

Janeane Bernstein, Ed.D. is a mental health advocate, journalist, and speaker. In response to the global pandemic, she created the mental health and wellness podcast and event series, *OUTSIDE THE BOX*. It includes her CARE Initiative, Creative Arts & Wellness Series, and other programming designed to address the mental health and wellness needs of students, teachers, and organizations of all sizes. She is the author of *Get the Funk Out!: %^&* Happens, What to Do Next!* in which she shares stories of resilience and the importance of prioritizing mental, physical, and emotional well-being. Bernstein hosts *Get the Funk Out!*, a weekly radio show on KUCI 88.9 FM.

She graduated from Syracuse University with a focus on communications and education and earned a doctorate from Boston University in Curriculum & Teaching. She is a 2021 Age Boom Academy Fellow with the Robert N. Butler Columbia Aging Center in partnership with Columbia Journalism.

Instagram: @otbseries @janeanebernstein
TikTok: @otbseries
www.otbseries.com
www.janeanebernstein.com